Ethical Dilemmas
in
Health Care

ETHICAL DILEMMAS

IN

HEALTH CARE

A Professional Search for Solutions

Edited by
Helen Rehr, D.S.W.

Published for The Doris Siegel Memorial Fund
of The Mount Sinai Medical Center
by PRODIST   New York   1978

Published for The Doris Siegel Memorial Fund
of The Mount Sinai Medical Center
by PRODIST
a division of
Neale Watson Academic Publications, Inc.
156 Fifth Avenue, New York 10010

Library of Congress Cataloging in Publication Data
Main entry under title:

Ethical dilemmas in health care.

    1.   Medical ethics—Congresses.   I.   Rehr,
Helen.   II.   Mount Sinai Medical Center.   [DNLM:
1.   Delivery of health care.   2.   Ethics, Medical.
W50.3 E84]
R724.E787   174′.2   78-17650
ISBN 0-88202-124-9

Designed and manufactured in U.S.A.

Man is as much influenced by natural forces as are other living things; but he constantly tries to escape from his biological bondage. For this reason, his future is shaped not only by the immutable and inexorable forces of nature, the effects of which are predictable, but even more by individual and collective decisions, which are largely unpredictable. The great moments of history are the new departures that result from these decisions. These are determined not by the *reactions* of the body machine, which are essentially passive, but by purposeful *responses*, which always imply choices. These responses are guided by man's ability to visualize the future, and indeed by his propensity to plan for a future which transcends his own biological life.

René Dubos, *A God Within*, p. 250
(With the kind permission of Charles Scribner's Sons)

Contents

Part 3   Conclusions

SAMUEL J. BOSCH
HELEN REHR
HAROLD LEWIS

Appendices

Preface

JANE BAERWALD ARON

It was an act of courage for The Doris Siegel Memorial Committee to select "Value and Ethical Dilemmas in the Delivery of Social Health Services" as the subject of its second colloquium, just as it was courageous to choose "Medicine and Social Work—An Exploration in Interprofessionalism" as the theme of its first. Each is a "first" in terms of formal public discussion by top practitioners in the field. Each is a fitting memorial to Doris Siegel.

Everything about Doris Siegel was a continuing lesson in courage. During her distinguished career in social work and particularly as Director of the Department of Social Service at The Mount Sinai Hospital, Doris worked for the best of social work in the classic sense, yet she boldly welcomed new ideas and herself initiated many of them. Under her aegis, the Social Service Department was among the first to include research as an integral component. In addition, it pioneered the Patient Services Representative (Ombudsman) as a vital part of the hospital's ambulatory care program, and it was on her initiative that the department reached out into the community before there was a Department of Community Medicine, or even before Mount Sinai School of Medicine was created.

Doris was a zealous advocate of professionalism in her department, but she was willing to share her knowledge and warm humanity with the lay members of the hospital "family." In this respect, her guidance and education of the Mount Sinai Auxiliary Board was an inspiring example of the mutual benefits to be derived from a "togetherness" of lay and professional.

When the first Chair in social work in an American medical school, the Edith J. Baerwald Professorship of Community Medicine (Social Work), was offered Doris at Mount Sinai School of Medicine, City University of New York, it took courage to say: "Yes, I'll tackle this." Many patients have benefitted from social work's part in medical education—the physician learned in his first year in medical school something about the social factors in health and illness and faced for the first time some of the ethical dilemmas and values involved in providing care to sick people.

With innate courage, Doris faced her illness and gave unstintingly of herself to the end of her life. Her many friends have therefore conceived of The Doris Siegel Memorial Fund as a living

1

memorial. It is the hope of the Memorial Fund Committee that these published proceedings will give added courage to the pioneers working for change in the delivery of social health services. And it is my personal hope that we in the lay community will have the courage to back them up. In the spirit of Doris Siegel, we are committed to moving forward in our mutual mission of providing the sick with professional skill and compassionate concern. These proceedings, we trust, will encourage that openness and courage which Doris bequeathed to all of us who were privileged to know and love her.

Jane Baerwald Aron
(Mrs. Jack R. Aron)
Vice Chairman of the Board
The Mount Sinai Medical Center

Introduction

HELEN REHR

In January 1976, The Doris Siegel Memorial Fund Committee (Appendix A) met to review its programmatic commitments to date and to project a second Doris Siegel memorial event. Suggestions to deploy income derived from the endowment fund included establishment of a scholarship to a medical student interested in social health issues, initiation of a visiting scholars' or great thinkers' program, or the exploration of a subject which could be covered in the same successful format as that of the first Doris Siegel Memorial Colloquium. During this exploratory session, the mission of The Doris Siegel Memorial Fund served as a constant reminder for excellence: "to encourage and support social work in its efforts to enhance the social effectiveness of health and medical care."

In concluding its discussion, the committee noted that by drawing from among the leaders of the three key health care professions—medicine, social work, and nursing—and by examining such an interprofessional interface the first colloquium had demonstrated that active participants could bring forth critical assessment, professional values, and interchange on the issue.[1] The committee then recommended that a timely subject be found and that selected health care professionals be given the opportunity to deliberate together, and to highlight their ideas, concepts, and contributions through the conference method and the subsequent publication of a monograph of the proceedings.

A subcommittee (Appendix B) was appointed and charged with identifying the most important current issue(s) relevant to social work and health care, the seminal leaders ready to deal with the issue(s), and the professional participants who could contribute substantively.

The subcommittee considered possible subjects over several months in 1976, always returning to the issue which identified the problem as centering around ethics and values in today's service organizations—the value dilemmas present in the health care climate. Those early deliberations touched on:

—the disappearance of the "social contract" in professionalism
—business as a dominant profession in hospitals, where medicine, nursing, and social work took a sub-ordered professional stance in

3

response to management and its expectations; management by objectives versus service based on needs

—the impact of federal funding patterns on the voluntary health care systems, and legislation dealing with charitable contributions or voluntary support

—the significance of pressures from multiple sources and the impact of these pressures and special interests on the values of the health care professionals

—securing accountability and quality assurance of the health care professionals and of the medical institution.

In the early discussion, the subcommittee identified the conflict that exists between the economic (efficiency and effectiveness) model and the humanistic model in health care delivery. It was suggested that values are translated into program planning and to a projection of ideological goals and objectives. When limited resources enter the picture, one can expect that allocation and "priority" demands would force "value" judgments in making choices. Furthermore, when choices have to be made, one can expect that social inequities and injustices will be introduced into the health care system. The subcommittee then struggled with the validity of a quality assurance system, trying to reconcile quality with professional values and ethics. The subject of quality assurance and value judgments raised such questions as: What should each profession measure? How is quality defined? By whom? Where in the service should quality be tested—in structure, process, or outcome? At what situation and when does one look for the effects of caring? Who measures those effects? Would the planning processes be affected? How does the situation impact on resources? How should resources be distributed into primary, preventive, secondary, and tertiary care?

This early topical consideration meant that we would have to examine: the kind of behaviors (by professionals) called for; the kind of knowledge required; how values are articulated into planning for programs; how they are integrated into interprofessional models of care; and how choices are made in regard to resource distribution.

In attempting to transform the subject into a program format, it was suggested that, in addition to prepared presentations, workshop groups involving selected invited participants would ask their members how values translate into ethics and goals. The groups would also look at behaviors in caring to determine whether an ethic is in evidence, and at the distribution of resources in terms of some

4

framework governing justice and equity. As we dealt with this approach, we realized the global nature of values and ethics in delivery and that the vagueness of values and the difficulty in defining them by the health professions contributed to the problem. We had wondered aloud whether a profession's existence is justified in relation to the standards, values, and ethics it professes.

As we acknowledged the difficulties in organizing the subject as a program, the subcommittee moved the discussion into a somewhat different context. We asked what questions are being raised in the health care field which are most significant, and how this group should raise them in the context of the Fund's objective of "the social effectiveness of health and medical care." Values began to emerge as we looked at the current emphases on efficiency, cost-effectiveness, and cost-containment on services and on their delivery. How do the social costs relate to the economic costs of programs? We suggested that, in recent projections, money and its availability has been the rationale for programming. Money has been used either as a hedge against change, as a negative social control, or in a positive sense of creative economics. We suggested that the most wasted resource is the human one, whether that of the professionals or the consumers. How do economic costs and social and human costs relate to each other? Too frequently, decision making in regard to allocation of funds for programs relfects the systems' abuse where the person in need is blamed and becomes the victim, while a system flourishes. The question of the true economics of health care was raised and examined in the context of its social consequences.

The subcommittee attempted to put some boundaries on the subject and finally entitled it: "Value and Ethical Dilemmas in the Delivery of Social Health Services." The subject was considered to cover policy, programs, and priorities as affected by efficiency expectation, the economics of the cost-effectiveness and cost-containment in services, and the meaning in relation to values and ethics in care. We asked: "Is there a relationship between economic and social costs in terms of social and human factors?"

One discussion by the subcommittee dealt with the codes of ethics that professions hold for themselves. In theory, professions are concerned with: (1) duties, (2) virtues, and (3) the common good. It was suggested that duties and virtues, (1) and (2), are more frequently related to than is the common good. This led to consideration of today's climate in the caring professions where there has

5

been indication of abrogating their "social contract." The "common good" was perceived in the tenet of the "right to care," rather than the "right to health." At this time the former was seen as feasible, the latter was not. It is recognized quickly that the "right to care" can be readily addressed under the frame of reference of the "Four A's": availability, accessibility, acceptability, and accountability. Each of the "A's" is affected by a wide range of factors: financing and payment methods; the culture of individuals; the costs of service and the inflationary spiral; the distribution and the allocation of resources; sectarian and special interests; the predilection of the planners, the policy and decision makers; institutional patterns and biases; professional expectations and preparation; consumer expectations; the leadership of the different health care professions; the mystique of medicine and the upward mobility and competitiveness of the other health care professions; manpower, its availability, its role allocation, and its distribution, its productivity and what each group has to offer; the responsibility of management and the influence of organized labor; the growing knowledge and better informed status of the public; the influence of the media; the utilization of services (who and what determines it), the meaning of and access to technological advances; the impact of malpractice claims and the growing defensiveness of medicine and other health care services. This discussion opened another series of issues which was seen as relevant: the personal responsibility of consumers and of providers, problems of equity versus distributive justice, the dichotomy between scientific and humanistic reasoning, and individualism versus the social good. The value and ethical imperatives in decision making arose as all of these factors were identified. "Who makes the decision? Who should make the decision? Who is affected and who is not?"

Once the subject was outlined in this way, the colloquium format became clearer and the identification of the keynoters comparatively simple. It was agreed that the keynote addresses should distinguish value and ethical dilemmas in delivery in the broad sense, in terms of economic costs and social costs. Two distinguished faculty members of the Mount Sinai School of Medicine[2] had each published on aspects of the subject from different perspectives. Dr. Victor Fuchs, currently at Stanford University, responded immediately in his willingness to return to Mount Sinai, where he had been Professor of Economics in Community Medicine, as well as at the Graduate School, both in the City University of New York. His earlier association with Doris Siegel was a major factor in his acquiescence. Mrs. Bess Dana, Associate Professor in the Department of Community Medicine, also agreed immediately to join Dr. Fuchs in addressing the subject. Mrs. Dana's ready commitment was lodged in a number of factors. First, she had been a professional colleague of Miss Siegel, having also been her student in their early Pittsburgh days. Second, Mrs. Dana has been a founding member of The Doris Siegel Memorial Committee, a seminal person in the design of the first colloquium, and responsible for a major chapter[3] in *Medicine and Social Work*, the proceedings of that event. Third, she and Dr. Fuchs had been associated in the educational program of the Department of Community Medicine and were thus natural partners. The subcommittee was most enthusiastic that the speakers on the first day of the colloquium would all be Mount Sinai faculty. The program format fell readily into place. These keynote speakers would be followed the next day by all-day workshop meetings in which the issues would be addressed by selected invited participants representing the three major health care professions plus others from law, economics, philosophy, the clergy, sociology, and administration. The workshop leaders in these fields would be drawn from government, practice, and education. They would be given a set of key concerns relative to the subject, and, having heard the speeches, would be expected to bring some resolution to issues and to suggest future direction for deliberation if resolution proved impossible.

The workshops were to be composed of individuals representing a mix of professions and disciplines. Response from the invited participants was excellent. The number of individuals who committed themselves to joining us moved us to expand the size of the workshops from the original ten participants, yet we attempted to safeguard the mix in order to permit diverse views to be expressed. Six groups of no more than fourteen each plus a leader and a recorder were finally agreed upon. As the planning developed further, the Brookdale Social Health Center for the Aging, represented by Drs. Helen Rehr and Richard Gorlin as co-principal investigators, proposed a seventh workshop which would address the same issues, but with reference to the elderly. All the invited participants of this group were experienced in the field of the aging and represented the same disciplines and professions as did the other invitees.

In preparing for the workshops, the subcommittee translated

7

the subject into specific issues to be addressed. The listing which was discussed with leaders and recorders one week before the working sessions and which was given to participants was as follows:

A. We are looking at value and ethical dilemmas in relation to the delivery of social health care. In that context:
1. Discuss the coexistence of societal needs and individual needs; the relationship of individual choice and self-determination to the broader common good and social equity; and the issues of availability and access.
2. Consider the impact of management prerogatives such as policy determination, productivity, et al.; professional and provider attitudes and behaviors, institutional design of medicine and hospitals; and other health care programs.
3. Address the issues of patients' rights and expectations; lifestyles, cultural attitudes and behaviors, and social-environmental resources in relation to compliance; utilization patterns; self-help as an economic or social choice.
4. Discuss the effects of the costs of care, financing patterns, fiscal arrangements, government interests, and other fiscal agents. Are cost-effectiveness and cost-benefit approaches compatible with social and humanistic values?
5. Address the impact of special interests; research expectations, touching on choice, availability, privacy, confidentiality, experimentation, costs, consent, et al.

B. Given the discussion regarding the issues, can be arrive at recommendations for health policies (federal and regional) dealing with:
1. Guarantees to access
2. Establishing priorities with respect to social health needs
3. Resource distribution and availability
4. Manpower levels, training, and distribution
5. Education affecting responsibilities, behavior, attitudes, and expectations of
   a. providers, and
   b. patients and families
6. Accountability for availability, quality, and cost-effectiveness.

The discussion of the guidelines with the leaders and the recorders noted that the items were not mandatory and that each group could deal with items as it wished. It was hoped that at least two issues of dilemmas would be addressed on the morning of May 6 and that, in the afternoon, some recommendations or directions for further deliberations on health policies would be arrived at.

Recorders were asked to be as detailed in their write-ups as they could and to have worked with the leaders in summarizing the discussions as soon after the workshops as possible. It was agreed that all would meet with Dr. Rehr in a feedback discussion of the proceedings for both general and specific reactions, and for content. The hope was that the written reports and the open discussion would serve as a section in the proceedings reflecting on the working parties' discussions.

The event was scheduled for the afternoon of May 5 and all day May 6, 1977, at The Mount Sinai Medical Center. The plenary session was attended by more than 550 persons including many friends of Doris Siegel, contributors to the Fund, directors of hospitals and members of their social work departments, deans of the schools of social work, representatives of selected health and social service agencies both public and voluntary, leaders from our East Harlem community, as well as individuals from all of The Mount Sinai Medical Center and of its affiliates, including members of both the Board of Trustees and the Auxiliary Board, administration, faculty, staff, the many professions of health care students, and the Social Work Services Departments of Mount Sinai, Beth Israel, Elmhurst, Joint Diseases, and Bronx VA Hospitals.

The Second Doris Siegel Memorial Colloquium was convened on May 5 by Dr. Helen Rehr, the Fund's Executive Secretary. She introduced Dr. Thomas C. Chalmers, Dean of Mount Sinai School of Medicine and President of The Mount Sinai Medical Center, who welcomed the audience. In addressing the group Dr. Chalmers also made reference to his lifelong professional commitment to "do clinical research, and to find that good clinical research is the best clinical care." He noted that we all face the challenge of examining what we do, so that we can do it better. The present state of knowledge in both the biomedical and the socioeconomic fields requires an ethical commitment to the assessment of what is done, and an examination of the results for recommendations and implementation of changes in practice as necessary. Dr. S. David Pomrinse followed with a special tribute to Doris Siegel. He commented on the subject of value and ethical dilemmas, noting Doris Siegel's special concern with the topic. Dr. Pomrinse also made reference to the currency of the subject and its difficulty for resolution, citing "the temper of the times, the political climate we live in, the emotional factors that drive us all, our various cultural heritages, religious experiences—. Trying to define out of this, or to

9

distill out of this complex series of things a clear message that all of us can agree with, a clear direction that all of us can follow, is inordinately difficult." He ended by noting that difficulties had never deterred Doris, nor Mount Sinai, and he believed that the speakers and participants would meet success in their efforts.

Dr. Kurt W. Deuschle, Chairman of the Department of Community Medicine and the Ethel H. Wise Professor, introduced Victor Fuchs and welcomed him back to Mount Sinai. Following his speech, Dr. Deuschle then introduced Bess Dana as the second speaker.

Dr. Fuchs' topic was "Values in Health" in which he addressed four issues:

1. Why try to place a value on health?
2. Can a value be placed on health?
3. Who determines the value of health? Who should determine the value?
4. Methods for estimating the value of health.

Dr. Fuchs immediately noted how emotionally laden the subject was, since it touched everyone, and each of us represented individual determinants and also the collective societal whole. Health maintenance is one of the most important goals in life. Yet it competes with other goals set by society for those scarce resources (such as land, labor, capital, time) which are available to us. Concern with health arises not only at the federal, state, and local governmental levels, but in both production and occupational climates in the private sector and in the philanthropic sector. The multidimensional aspects of health touching on life expectancy, disability and its relationship to physical and social functioning, pain and illnesses, treatment choices and risks, costs of care and procedures, age-related illnesses and disabilities make it even more difficult to put values on health. Yet we do put values on it all the time, whether in providing Medicare and Medicaid programs, public health legislation, or even in setting speed limits to serve as accident deterrents. All of us, he suggested, make decisions about health at some time; government regulators, administrators, politicians, and providers make them for us most of the time. He posed the key question of what influences people's choices and recognized the influence of special interests. He asked the members of the audience if each could be a "disinterested party" with regard to choices and decisions about health, reminding us that rational decisions are ideal, but difficult. He admonished us to "beware of experts" since their value judgments are no better than those of "people—all of us." Dr. Fuchs cited the difficulty of measuring the value of health and suggested that evaluation be placed at the system level where choice and rationing should take place, insulating the individual practitioner within the system of care. The clinician, he believed, must be system-rational and accountable therein. He suggested that the preventive health behavior which medicine has pressed for has met failure because of the uncertainty of the health effects and he himself sees such behavior as really "only changes in the probability" of outcome. In any case, he said, he could not answer why society does not behave rationally. He concluded by saying that values in judgment must be tempered by humanistic spirit and hardheadedness.

Mrs. Bess Dana's topic was "Value Dilemmas in the Delivery of Social Health Services: Caring, Coping, and Curing." Mrs. Dana noted that she had been asked to discuss the subject "from the point of view of social justice and equity in relation to social choice and resource availability in the delivery of social health care."[4]

Mrs. Dana opened her talk by suggesting she would not let clinicians off the hook of value judgments in relation to care. Daily feedback from practice can help us make value choices. Evaluation cannot be limited to the system level alone but must be viewed at the individual practitioner's level as well. She viewed "help and helping" as the operational expression of social justice and equity. Helping guides the value measures by reflecting the distance the helper will go in bridging the gap between help and helplessness in some people. She cited the inconsistencies in believing that independence, freedom of choice, and self-determination exist while disregarding the relationship of social choice and social opportunity. On the other side, she noted that use and utilization patterns of people reflect their abuse and place responsibility on the consumer as well. She believes that, under the pressure for cost control, the first services to be dropped are the humanistic support programs. Value is placed on self-reliance and on compliance by those in the health services. This value is held for those populations which are at special risk such as the elderly, the handicapped, the poor who frequently possess less resources and are often without voice in health care determinants. While we constantly hold to the axiom of "helping people help themselves," she believes interdependence of human beings and services is the value need for people "at risk."

She stated that the major health problems today are those

which are chronic and long-term and not acute, i.e., those which can be controlled, not cured. Most health care needs are dependent on long-term investments in caring by providers and in coping by the recipient. The investment in securing positive end goals is more dependent on factors and programs touching social-psychological interventions and not limited to those in the biomedical establishment. The scientific and technological resources of the hospital represent only one aspect of care. Prevention of disease and maintenance of health must be looked at more in ecological and environmental causes and effects as well as in biomedical terms. In her opinion a bio-psycho-social model which includes a social support system would meet today's social health needs far better than the present day biomedical care model. The awareness of personal, industrial, occupational, environmental, and family life-styles must underpin any system of care. Interdependence between patient, therapist, and program of care, rather than independence and self-help alone should be the optimum tenet in health care programs. She endorsed interprofessionalism as the primary interventive style, with emphasis on developing primary care along with secondary and tertiary care programs. It was Mrs. Dana's opinion that the only moral ground for discrimination in services is the degree of need presented by different groups. Finally, she held each profession to the values and ethics of its social contract with the public; these, she believes, remain consistent principles to be followed no matter to whom they are applied.

The working parties, which met throughout the following day, initiated their discussion with emphasis on values and ethics governing the professions which provide health care services. The participants were divided into seven groups, of which six had the same working agenda, and the seventh was to use the agenda with special reference to the elderly. The discussants came from the health care professions as well as from law, economics, philosophy, sociology, administration, and the clergy (Appendix C). All were known for their contributions to health care and related fields, and represented government, practice, and/or education. Except for those who had specialized in the field of aging (representing the same range of professions and disciplines) and who met in their own workshop, the others were randomly assigned to the six groups. The assignments were made to assure that non-health care professions were represented in each of the workshops.

Each of the workshops had its own leader and recorder. All the leaders and recorders met prior to the colloquium for a briefing on the objectives of the discussion groups. There were two such briefing sessions, based on guidelines prepared by the planning subcommittee (Appendix B). Each of the briefing sessions became a working party in itself, producing points of view on value and ethical dilemmas in practice and in programs.

The discussions of the working parties are analyzed in Part II. The analysis derives from the briefing sessions, the minutes of each workshop as reviewed by the workshop leader, and from the follow-up "feedback" sessions. In addition, the planning subcommittee members "floated" through the seven workshops and met later to review the entire colloquium proceedings.

Before bringing this introduction to its conclusion, it is important to recognize that an event of this moment and magnitude requires a host of people to organize and implement it, and to bring to fruition its proceedings, and I would like to acknowledge our gratitude to all of them. First, I want to express our deep appreciation to the Brookdale Social Health Center on the Aging at the Mount Sinai Medical Center in their support of the workshop on aging. The special paper prepared by Drs. Gideon Horowitz and John Maher represents the work of workshop members committed to serving this population. As you read the papers of Dr. Fuchs and Mrs. Dana, you will see how meaningful their contributions are to the subject, and were to the discussion of the workshop participants. Dr. Samuel Bosch, joined by Dr. Rehr, assumed responsibility for the most difficult task: synthesizing the reports, the feedback sessions of leaders and recorders, and the subcommittee which resulted in the chapter "A Professional Search into Values and Ethics in Health Care Delivery." Dr. Harold Lewis agreed to join with Drs. Bosch and Rehr to address conclusions and recommendations, and these are found in the final chapter, entitled "Some Suggested Remedies, Resolutions, and Further Deliberations." I want to comment on the extraordinary nature of this subcommittee. In addition to planning and implementing the colloquium, the members mentioned above, and Mrs. Bea Phillips, Dr. Maurice Russell, Mrs. Elinor Stevens, and Mrs. Dana have stamped these final proceedings with their analyses which took place in a meeting the first week in July, and resulted in their commitment to its writing. We are indebted to Helen Bronheim who edited these proceedings. All of the subcommittee is to be commended for its tireless efforts in making the plenary session, the workshops, and the social events as successful as they proved to be.

Mrs. Marjorie Pleshette staffed and coordinated all aspects of the colloquium and the proceedings. I believe that without Marjorie none of this "show" would have seen the light of day. She had the invaluable assistance of Mrs. Margery Levenstein and members of the Auxiliary Board. Mrs. Robert M. Benjamin, lay member of the Subcommittee on Planning and a long-time friend to social work and Doris, again opened her home in extraordinary hospitality to our out-of-town guests and members of The Doris Siegel Memorial Committee. The staff at Mount Sinai, not only those of the Department of Social Work Services, but so many others contributed generously toward making the event so positive an experience for so many.

Helen Rehr, D.S.W.
Director, Department of Social Work Services
The Mount Sinai Hospital
Edith J. Baerwald Professor of Community Medicine (Social Work)
Mount Sinai School of Medicine
City University of New York

References

[1] *Medicine and Social Work: An Exploration in Interprofessionalism*, edited by Helen Rehr. New York: PRODIST, 1974.
[2] Victor R. Fuchs, *Who Shall Live? Health, Economics and Social Choice*. New York: Basic Books Inc., 1974.
Bess Dana, "The Social Components of Health Care Systems," *Encyclopedia of Social Work*. New York, National Association of Social Workers, Inc., 1977.
[3] Bess Dana, H. David Banta, and Kurt W. Deuschle "Part 3 Conclusions and Recommendations: An Agenda for the Future of Interprofessionalism," *Medicine and Social Work*, edited by Helen Rehr. New York: PRODIST, 1974.
[4] From Dr. Rehr's letter of invitation, as suggested by the subcommittee.

Part 1
The Working Papers

Values in Health:
An Economist's Perspective[1]

VICTOR R. FUCHS

The "value" of health is a subject laden with emotion and fraught with conceptual and measurement problems. It is also the object of political controversy and you may well question why I would approach such a subject. Some of you are probably thinking "He is very brave;" some are probably thinking "He is very foolish;" and by the time I have finished some of you may think I am both. I think this is an important topic and I will address it somewhat in the spirit of Passover—that is, I will ask and try to answer four questions:

First, why try to place a value on health? Second, can a value be placed on health? Third, who determines, or who should determine, the value of health? And fourth, how can the value of health be measured?

First: Why place a value on health? Isn't health so much more important than anything else in life that it would be impossible to place a value on it? An ancient proverb says "He who has health has hope, and he who has hope has everything." Obviously a human life is priceless; therefore how can you possibly put a price on it?

But that is precisely what I am going to talk about. And the fundamental reason we need to talk about these questions is because health competes with other goals at every level of society. Some of the other goals are quite noble: justice, truth, beauty. Some are a little more mundane: creature comforts, pleasures. But these other goals do compete with health for the scarce resources of society. They compete for land, for labor, for capital, for our time, energy, and attention. This competition can be observed in the federal budget: health now takes some $50 billion, but it competes with national defense, energy research, and other priorities.

At the state and local levels, health also competes with other demands, education being a prime example. In the world of philanthropy there are foundations and philanthropists who are completely committed to health; others are not; still others are trying to make judgments about the value of committing resources to health as opposed to committing them elsewhere. In the business world and in the production of various goods, there are health hazards associated with various production processes, and choices

17

have to be made. Shall we change the process? How much will it cost to change it? What value accrues if we make the change? At the level of the individual and the family, we constantly make choices which affect our health, what we do, what we consume, how we live. Implicitly we are making valuations—judgments about the worth of change opposed to what we must sacrifice or spend.

There is another reason which underscores the complexity of the problem—the multidimensional aspects of health. Health is not just one thing. It may be life expectancy: Will a person live? Will s/he die? How long will s/he live? Health could be a question of disability, of not being able to function as well as one wishes. It may be a question of pain and suffering; it may be a question of illness. In addition, there are the questions concerning *who* is sick or *whose* life expectancy we are talking about. Is it a young child? An old person? And there are differing dimensions to diseases. Are we talking about ill health resulting from heart disease or cancer? Accidents? Because of these multidimensional factors it becomes even more important and more difficult to place values on varying states of health.

Suppose there are two ways of treating a seriously ill person. One is a radical procedure with a 40 percent chance of death, but a 60 percent chance of full recovery and a normal life. A second, less radical treatment carries a 10 percent chance of death, a 30 percent chance of full recovery, and a 60 percent chance of survival with partial disability. Let us assume that the procedures are equal in cost. Which should be followed? The question cannot be answered unless one is prepared to place values on the alternative health outcomes. Something else to think about: Would your answer be different if one procedure is ten times costlier than the other? Should that change the choice in relationship to the values?

There are also age dimensions. People suffer from different things at different points in life. Young children and premature infants need different kinds of health care than do adults; some people need organ transplants or renal dialysis. These considerations complicate the problem, but far from providing reasons for *not* trying, they make even more compelling the need for fixing values. It becomes a matter of ethical responsibility to "value" if we are to make ethically responsible decisions and choices, since these situations will always be with us and it is obvious we cannot do everything for everyone.

It is essential to understand that this necessity for choice is not related to the fact that we live in a money economy, although values may be denoted in money terms. It is not related to the fact that we live in a capitalist society or that we live in an industrial society. The necessity for choices exists in all societies and under all kinds of regimes. In Communist China they have to make choices—they can't treat every health problem, so they have a valuation process that tells them they want to treat this health problem rather than that one. Robinson Crusoe on his island may have seen some nice fruit at the top of a tall tree. He had to judge whether the fruit was worth the risk of falling from the tree and breaking an arm or a leg. All of these are valuation problems connected with allocation decisions.

The second question to be considered is "Can we put a value on health?" My answer is simple: "We do, all the time." We implicitly do so every time we make decisions about resources which have health implications. If a community decides to put up a traffic light at a school crossing (or not to put up a traffic light) they have made a decision involving implicit valuation of health. If we raise the speed limit from 55 to 65 miles per hour (or if we don't), there is a valuation implicit in that choice.

In the administration of a hospital, in the decision to build a hospital, expand (or not expand) a hospital, health valuations are constantly being made. Whichever way the decision goes, a value is being put on health, up or down.

Sometimes these decisions are made explicitly, but more often they are made implicitly. Who should make these valuations? Who *does* make these valuations? This difficult question is partly answered by what I have already said: People make these valuations—people in legislative bodies, in government regulatory agencies, and in administrations of non-profit institutions. Individuals make these valuations by choices in their own lifestyles, in the way they choose to live and work.

Can ethically justifiable decisions be made in the public policy area? Understandably, each group will push for the values and health problems that concern it. Parents of crippled children will attach a high value to assistance to crippled children. People who need organ transplants will say that these should have high priority. Those who have had a stroke and need rehabilitation will want that area emphasized.

How can one approach this in a neutral or ethical spirit? One possibility is the "device of the original position" used by Harvard

19

philosopher John Rawls in his book *A Theory of Justice*. Imagine, says Rawls, that you didn't know who you were going to be on Earth, that this decision you were participating in was to take place before you were born and you had no idea of your relative position in life. Imagine that you are able to influence how the resources will be allocated and how the values will be established. What kinds of values would you choose then? Where would you have society put its resources? How much emphasis should it give to one thing as opposed to another?

Since your decisions are reached from a completely disinterested position, you would presumably approach them in a rational manner. You might reason that going through life will mean exposure to this and that condition and that it would seem sensible for society to attempt to care for certain ones. This would mean putting values on various health outcomes.

One of the things I would like to emphasize throughout this decision about valuation is to beware of experts. Experts are useful people to have around to tell you technical things. You need experts if you want to know, for example, the kind of health effect you might get from a particular type of medical intervention, or from a particular change in behavior, such as stopping smoking or beginning to exercise. But when it comes to placing a value on the projected outcome (how much it is worth to do this or that), my values tell me to beware of experts. The people affected should have the greatest say in how it should be valued.

I offer a simple example of this which crossed my desk the other day in the form of a "health risk analysis report" put out by Serle. This is a computer analysis of the patient's history, test results, behavior, etc., in relation to what is known about how these inputs are likely to affect the patient's health (in this particular case, life expectancy). Here's a man 35 years old whose life expectancy is projected on the basis of his history, blood pressure, and other inputs. The analysis shows him the kind of change in life expectancy he could expect were he to follow a variety of prescriptive or proscriptive actions with varying values attached.

I don't know how accurate these analyses are, nor am I recommending that approach. However, I *am* pointing out an alternative to the authoritarian doctor pounding the desk, ordering certain courses of action and forbidding certain others. It can become a matter of pointing out, "Here are the best judgments on the possible consequences of various courses of action. Now you,

Mr. Patient, rank-order the values. You decide whether the probable outcomes are worth it to you, given what is required of you."

Of course there may be decisions where, from an economic point of view, it would not be socially optimal to allow individual decision making to prevail. Those are cases of externalities where the behavior of certain individuals has implications for other individuals and there is no way of effecting a compensation one way or the other. Vaccination is a good example of an externality with a "public good" aspect; pollution is an example of an externality which creates a "public bad" aspect. In those cases we would use governmental mechanisms (particularly subsidies and taxes) to influence people's behavior to be more consistent with what would be socially desirable.

Now we come to another difficult question: How do we actually get measures of the value of health and place dollar values on it? To date there are several different approaches, but none is really satisfactory. I offer a few in the spirit of example—the base from which we start and try to do better.

One of the best known approaches is to look, not directly at the value of health, but at the opposite side of the coin, the cost of illness. In developing this approach Barbara Cooper and Dorothy Rice have analyzed the cost of illness for people of different ages for different kinds of diseases. Costs are broken down into three categories: (1) the direct cost of illness (the medical cost, hospital cost, drug cost, etc.); (2) costs of morbidity, which are measured primarily in terms of foregone earnings and the foregone services of housewives; and (3) mortality cost, which again is done in terms of foregone services.

This kind of approach is instructive. For one thing, it gives some notion of the value of health by looking at the negative side—that not being healthy is being sick. It also permits a look at the value of reductions in various diseases. As you might imagine, the figures vary depending upon whether you're simply counting the number of people who died from a particular disease, or whether you're using a dollar value approach as Cooper and Rice do—looking at future earnings and applying some rate of discount in an effort to derive a dollar value.

Let me give you one striking result. If you survey deaths from various causes you'll find that 53 percent of all deaths in the United States in 1972 were from diseases of the circulatory system and only 8 percent of deaths were due to accidents or violence of various types. But if you apply their valuation technique and ask what percentage of the cost of all deaths is accounted for by these two causes, circulatory diseases account for 32 percent while accidents and violence account for 25 percent. In other words, measured only in lives there is a sixfold difference in importance between the two causes, but according to one widely used system of valuation, the two causes are not far from equal in importance.

The reason for this, of course, is the ages of the different people involved, since accidents and violence kill proportionately more people in the younger and middle ages, while circulatory diseases take their toll at much older ages.

You may not like the values Cooper and Rice used; you may think they're wrong; you may quarrel with their methods, even granting their approach; or you may point out that they don't put in a value for "pain and suffering," for example. Admittedly there are many ways they could be criticized, but my point is that *something* must be done. If you have criticism you should speak up, but you should be prepared to show why this isn't the right way, and what would be a better way.

Let me mention just a couple of other instances. Some of my colleagues decided to examine the question of valuation of life by looking at occupations with varying risk attached, ascertaining the wages paid in these occupations, and inferring the valuation from the differentials in wages. In other words: If you take two men of the same schooling, age, and other characteristics, but observe one in an occupation with considerable risk and the other in a less hazardous occupation, you will likely see a differential in earnings. This was to be done systematically over several thousand workers in an effort to tease out an implicit valuation to be assigned the differential risks of workers collectively through the workings of the labor market. The result is a total, implicit value of life which is not too different from the one Cooper and Rice arrived at using their discounted future earnings approach.

Let me mention one more type of evidence: jury awards. As you know, juries are composed of ordinary people, not experts. They have to sit and listen to the evidence that a person's health has been impaired by malpractice or by an accident. They are then expected to place a value on that event. Juries cannot ignore this issue nor say they cannot value human life. They must, and do, put a value on human life.

22

Two of my students have been studying jury awards in malpractice cases in California and have been ascertaining the values people place on life. One of their findings in cases resulting in death is that values placed on life at different ages follow essentially the age-value profile which emerges from the Cooper-Rice approach of discounted future earnings. Where the result was severe injury rather than death, jury awards do not follow this age-profile valuation scheme. We surmise that this is because the juries are awarding money for future medical care costs, for pain and suffering, and for other considerations which go beyond loss of future earnings.

Another interesting development in jury awards stands in contrast to the Cooper-Rice approach: In the jury awards examined, there was no systematic difference between awards to men and awards to women. Juries apparently recognize that although women's earnings in the labor market are lower than those of men, there is another aspect to be considered—that which we economists call the non-market production function (the value of what the woman contributes in the home without pay). Juries are apparently awarding (given the severity of injury or illness) about the same for both sexes.

These are examples of valuation techniques—none of them perfect, none even very good. (Bob Hutchins, former Chancellor of the University of Chicago, was fond of saying that it was not a very good university, but it was the best there was.) To value or not to value: that is *not* the question. Rather, the question is to value explicitly, systematically, democratically—or to value implicitly, haphazardly, autocratically. It is useless to pretend the sky is the limit—that we can do everything possible for health; that we can do everything possible to save human life. That is fiction and has always been fiction. If we pursue that delusion we will become expansive, only to be forced to cut back sharply, thus perpetuating the wild swings and contortions that have plagued the health field in recent years.

In conclusion, I would say the emphasis for us (and perhaps for some of your discussions tomorrow) should be on how to improve the valuation process, and on how we can insulate the individual practitioner—social worker, physician, or another working in a one-to-one situation—where such valuation is inappropriate and contrary to the spirit of the particular situation. I am not saying that valuation occurs at that level; rather, that valuation occurs at the system level where decisions are being made about resource utilization: what resources will be available, what procedures will be followed, what standards will obtain, etc.

We need to be considering how the individual practitioner can appreciate the need for system valuation and system rationing, and at the same time be insulated from it at least in the immediate environment, given the constraints. These are difficult things to achieve; difficult to talk about—but that is the challenge. Mount Sinai is a great medical center. It is a center that has made great contributions toward the cure of disease and the treatment of sick people. It is my hope that it will also pioneer in these new difficult areas, bringing to bear upon these problems both a humanistic spirit and the hardheadedness needed to do the very best possible in what will always be a difficult choice.

Victor R. Fuchs, PH.D.
Director
Center for Economic Analysis of Human Behavior and Social Institutions
Stanford, California

Reference

[1] The helpful comments of Claire Gilchrist are gratefully acknowledged.

Value Dilemmas in the Delivery of Social Health Services: Caring, Coping, and Curing

BESS DANA

Introduction

For me, participation in today's tribute to Doris Siegel represents in many ways the continuation of a process set in motion in Doris' office in Pittsburgh's Montefiore Hospital some thirty years ago. It was there, as a second-year student in social work, that I first began to confront the almost daily—and *always* painful—necessity for reconciling personal, professional, and societal values as the unremitting demand of professionalism. I count myself fortunate indeed to have been first alerted to the power of health care issues to continuously shake up intellectual and moral postures and to alter concepts of self in relation to the health needs and problems of others by a teacher who managed at one and the same time to be softhearted and tough-minded. For Doris, healing the breach between science and humanism was a lifetime pursuit and the goal she transmitted to all of us who knew her as a teacher, practitioner, and friend.

I have been asked—and I quote directly from Dr. Rehr's letter of invitation to me on behalf of the Doris Siegel Memorial Committee—"to discuss value dilemmas in the delivery of social health services from the point of view of social justice and equity in relation to social choice and resource availability in the delivery of social health care." In reducing the enormity of this charge to the scale of my own knowledge, experience, values, and not inconsiderable bias, I have elected to talk about help and helping as the operational expressions of the freedom and constraints which our interpretations of social justice impose on man's responsibility for man.

Defining Social Health Services

Social health services, in the context of this paper, represent then the degree of responsibility that society accepts, at any given time, for supporting and supplementing personal resources for dealing

25

with the demands inherent in maintaining health, preventing disease, and caring for, coping with, and curing illness. Social health services are thus greatly influenced in substance, in delivery style, in scope and coverage, by the value judgments that we as a society employ in justifying or sanctioning dependency, the degree and duration of dependency we are willing to tolerate—and under what circumstances—and our behavioral expectations from the dependent—by way of gratitude, compliance, investment and divestment of economic, sociocultural, and psychological holdings.

Helping represents these value judgments converted into action. As such, it is a measure of the distance we are willing to go in bridging the gap between *help* and *helplessness*. The meaning that Webster ascribes to each term provides a useful guide in estimating the breadth of the gap to be traversed. According to Webster, *help* is activity designed: *"(1)* to make it easier for (a person) to *(a)* do something; aid; assist—specifically *(b)* to give something necessary; *(c)* to do part of the work or share the labor; *(2)* to make it easier for something to exist, happen, develop, improve; *(3)* to cause improvement; remedy; improve." *Helplessness*, as defined by Webster, indicates a state or condition of being *"(1)* without power to help oneself, feeble, weak; *(2)* without help or protection; *(3)* incompetent; inefficient; *(4)* irremediable."

By standard definition then, help and helplessness are value-laden terms—and, as such, defy an absolute interpretation. The seemingly subtle gradations in meaning that Webster ascribes to them are magnified in their translation into the language of everyday life where they appear as inconsistencies in existing health and medical care policies and practices and/or as opposing positions in the continuing debate regarding the appropriate balance between individual and social responsibility along the whole continuum from health maintenance through disease prevention, treatment, and control. Is it, for instance, the threat of uncontrolled costs, of systems abuse, of "watering down" the quality of medical care that are the principal motivating factors that deter us, time after time, from the aggressive pursuit of the removal of financial barriers to access to medical care as national health policy and provision? Or does our wavering action reflect the unresolved question as to whether help—i.e., "to assist, to give something necessary"—stifles or frees the individual capacity for independence and self-sufficiency as the ultimate expression of the American ethic? Is this same distrust of helping as a hedge against helplessness expressed in the inescapable fact that support services are the first items to be scratched in both public and voluntary efforts to achieve cost control, cost containment, and cost reduction in health care? How, except through acknowledgment of our value dissonance, do we reconcile our encouragement of helplessness, passivity, compliance as attributes of the "good" hospital patient with our implicit or explicit honoring of self-responsibility and resourcefulness upon hospital discharge—or, for that matter, in seeking medical care initially?

Does our seeming inability to find creative ways to stretch our helping reach to encompass the needs of the growing population of the chronically ill, those among the aged who, in fact, are "without power to help themselves"—"feeble"; "weak"; "without help or protection"; many times legally "incompetent;" and too often still, "irremediable"—reflect limitations in our intellectual and material resources? Or is the failure to provide comprehensive social health services to the aged and chronically sick without "power to help themselves" further evidence of our inability to come to social health terms with the full meaning of the help-helplessness connection?

Caring, Coping, and Curing Revisited

These and related questions have nagged at the conscience of American society since our beginning as an independent nation. At an abstract level, they reflect the essential tension inherent in the concept of democracy itself, with the necessity it imposes to contain individual freedom and independence within the constraints of law and equity as protectors and guardians of the common good. Far from receding as central issues with our burgeoning scientific knowledge and technological proficiency, the value dilemmas associated with the formulation of social health policy and its implementation in the delivery of social health services have become increasingly convoluted, acute, and resistant to quick resolution almost—or so it seems—with every new scientific breakthrough and/or technological advance. Equity in the pre-scientific era was easier to achieve when there were fewer benefits to be distributed; compassion easier to evoke in the care of the sick when it was the major instrumentality in the physician's armamentarium; and dependency less to be feared when illness itself was short-term in nature, its outcome either full recovery or death.

27

Maintaining health, preventing, caring for, coping with, and curing illness present, in our time, significantly different tasks and responsibilities from those early days when many of the values that still persist in our present-day perception of individual versus social responsibility in health and illness originated. The nature of illness itself—its natural history, course, and consequences—has altered in several important ways:

— Infectious disease, once the principal agent of mortality and morbidity, has been virtually conquered, only to be replaced by illnesses of long duration, with their differential demands on individual and social resources.

— Salient features of the chronic diseases as they influence social health needs and interventions include both their long latency periods and their association with social and psychological as well as biological risk factors. (Put another way, the forces that make and keep people sick begin their insidious attack long before the appearance of overt signs and symptoms of disease and are recruited from such diverse sources as genetic endowment, habits and circumstances of daily living, conditions of the physical and work environment, personal pleasures, indulgences, and deprivations.)

— Chronic disease, in contrast to infectious disease, lends itself at our present level of knowledge and understanding more readily to containment than to cure. Curing, when it is in fact possible, is more and more dependent on a long-time investment in caring and in coping.

Indeed, it becomes increasingly difficult to identify a single modern advance—whether in the prevention, control, or conquest of disease—that does not make significant and continuing demands on the coping and caring capacities of patient and family, or that does not depend for its successful implementation on the continuing availability of and access to a wide and diverse range of technological and professional services and psycho-social, economic, and environmental supports. It is precisely this comprehensive and continuous demand that caring for, coping with, and solving contemporary health problems makes on personal, professional, and social resources that brings into sharp focus the relationship between health and social opportunity and links the cause of health with social equity and social justice. Our accumulating evidence about the characteristics of the population at highest risk for the major chronic illnesses serves to underscore these connections:

28

He or she who gets sick or is most threatened by sickness in America today is more likely to be poor or near poor than affluent; he or she is more likely to be non-white than white; to have less formal educaton than his or her healthier peers; to live in poorer housing; to eat more empty calories; to drink more alcohol, smoke more cigarettes, abuse more drugs; and to have less access to primary and secondary medical care—in other words, to experience and express, in the aggregate, the whole dreary litany of social, economic, and psychological deprivation that at one and the same time predisposes to physical and mental breakdown and militates against recovery.

Social Health Versus Biomedical Needs and Interventions

Whether defined in terms of the characteristics of the population at highest risk for disease or the particular disease entities that pose the greatest threat to the health of Americans, today's health problems can obviously no longer be contained within what Engel[1] terms the "neat and tidy" boundaries of the biomedical model nor solved by the resources of the biomedical establishment alone. Giving up this model, which has for over half a century profoundly influenced personal, professional, and institutional thought and action in health and disease, has the consequence of forcing professional and public confrontation with medical and social realities which the biomedical model has tended to obscure, ignore, or protect against: i.e., the fact of the long-term nature of disease itself with all that implies by way of actual or potential loss of personal freedom and control; the limitations in the capacity of science and technology to control, modify, or eradicate major life-threatening illnesses; the social costs and consequences of unattended personal and family problems associated with illness and its management; the unmet needs of the walking sick and the worried well; the inequitable allocation and distribution of biomedical benefits and services among various segments of the population defined by such variables as age, sex, ethnicity, socioeconomic status, diagnosis, or stage of illness.

For provider and consumer alike, acting on new perceptions of reality as illuminated by epidemiological and behavioral science research, clinical observations, and practice wisdom poses serious threats to the balance of power among the people, the professions,

29

and health and medical care institutions; raises the complicated questions of health as a social choice that Dr. Fuchs[2] has so clearly explicated; and challenges the values of freedom and autonomy that both the people and the professions hold so dear. For whatever its limitations—and they are many—the biomedical model of health care delivery provides a means of legitimizing dependency on the basis of objective physical findings that a social health delivery model, with its considerations of subjective as well as objective data as evidence of need, does not. The biomedical model provides clear guidelines for the determination of personal and professional responsibilities in health and medical care that a social health delivery model tends to blur. And, in a curious way, through its very neglect of the social components of health and disease, the biomedical model offers more freedom from social controls on both, personal and professional autonomy than is likely to be possible under a social health frame of reference for defining and dealing with health problems.

Expanding the boundaries of health and medical care to accommodate the territorial requirements of social and psychological phenomena therefore involves more than intellectual acceptance of the part that these phenomena play in the cause, course, and outcome of illness. If health and medical care services are to allow for the full expression of social health wants and provide full attention to social health needs, both the public and the health care establishment (professions and institutions) must acknowledge and work through what Fowler[3] terms "the twentieth century dilemma," i.e., the requirement "to pay in terms of personal freedom for the contempt felt at the absence of social freedom." Since the mid-sixties, the effort—both public and professional—to deal more aggressively with this dilemma as expressed in the substance, scope, and delivery style of health care services has accelerated, spurred on initially by the more general human rights movement, and, in more recent times, by the need to stem the runaway costs of health and medical care:

> —Helping people help themselves—that old social work maxim—now applied to population groups in the community as well as patients and patient groups in medical care facilities, reveals untapped strengths and resources within consumers, their indigenous self-help systems, and their communities that, with appropriate professional and techni-

cal reinforcement, can be engaged as essential components of the health care system already in place.

—Primary care viewed in the Rogers[4] terms as a "coping system," particularly when it is incorporated within a prepaid group practice model, acts as an effective means of fortifying the coping and caring capacities of patients and families and at the same time deterring the inappropriate use of diagnostic and treatment facilities.

—Preventive interventions in the form of support systems located where the problems are—the work place, the neighborhood health center, the school—have already begun to show significant success in helping people overcome such adverse health behavior as smoking, alcohol abuse, and overeating and in adhering to hypertension control regimens.

Out of these small but steady efforts to join the resources of the health professions and institutions with the resources of the people in a redefinition of rights and responsibilities *in* and *to* health care, a persuasive case begins to emerge for giving up our spoken or unspoken fears about the damaging effects of helping on self-reliance and independence and moving more surefootedly toward: (1) *the acceptance of interdependence as the operative value for the organization and delivery of social health services*; and (2) *the revitalization of interprofessionalism as our interventive mode.*

As members of the health professions—whether physicians, nurses, social workers, or research scientists—we constitute part of a bruised society. Whether rightly or wrongly, our professional image has been shattered, our integrity seriously questioned. We need from each other both intellectual stimulation and emotional reinforcement in order to respond with the full engagement of our collective knowledge, skills, and compassionate commitment to the demanding scientific, technical, economic, and deeply human problems of health care delivery in these unsettled times.

In tribute then to Doris Siegel—that remarkable warmhearted and tough-minded woman who accepted fully the interactive nature of giving and receiving help, I would urge that we

—acknowledge in our social health action that the gap between help and helplessness is experienced unequally among different population groups in this society;

—apply in social health policy and services Campbell's[5] principle that the only moral ground for discrimination is the degree of need presented by different groups and individuals; and

—maintain in our professional practices what Frankel[6] terms "the supreme moral duty of all professions: a willingness to make choices in terms of the facts as they can best be established, and in terms of principles that remain consistent no matter to whom they are applied."

Bess Dana, M.S.S.A.
Associate Professor
Director, Education Unit
Department of Community Medicine
Mount Sinai School of Medicine
City University of New York

References

[1] George L. Engel, "The Need for a New Medical Model: A Challenge for Biomedicine," *Science* (April 8, 1977): 129–136.

[2] Victor R. Fuchs, *Who Shall Live? Health, Economics, and Social Choice.* New York: Basic Books, 1974.

[3] John Fowler, *Daniel Martin.* Boston: Little, Brown & Company, 1977, p. 260.

[4] David E. Rogers, "The Challenge of Primary Care," *Daedalus* (Winter 1977): 81ff.

[5] A.V. Campbell, "Establishing Ethical Priorities in Medicine," *British Medical Journal* (1977): 818–821.

[6] Charles Frankel, "Social Values and Professional Values," *Education for Social Work* (Spring 1969): 33.

Part 2
The Working Parties

A Professional Search into Values and Ethics in Health Care Delivery

HELEN REHR

SAMUEL J. BOSCH

Preface

The difficulty of the subject was acknowledged by all participants in the day-long workshops; many were frustrated and pained by a perceived failure to resolve these issues. Yet no one left the group experience affectively untouched. In the aftermath of the workshops, one heard "stimulating," "exciting," "frustrating," "good participation," "fascinating ideas." The group process served to give heart to each participant and a feeling of emerging from the isolation of grappling with these concerns alone by learning of what was going on in the world outside their own domains. While frustration, discouragement, and struggle against constraints were voiced, they were subject-ordered and not related to the group process itself.

The mix of professions and disciplines was viewed as highly stimulating, permitting many ideas to emerge, albeit with problems. While in most instances the professional backgrounds served to make the content specific, it was the personality of the participants that was most meaningful. The groups were made up of "stars," "experts," each of whom saw his or her "mission" as that of communicating his own point of view. Although many of the members knew or knew of each other, they had not interrelated in a group before. With such a limited amount of time for discussion, it was almost impossible to reach group consensus in most of the areas, and very little was achieved in the way of resolution. There was never the intention that consensus on issues need be found. Certainly, the diversity of backgrounds among the participants contributed to the groups' inability to reach common accord. That diversity also contributed to the richness of the discussion. In addition there was early recognition that the subject is in itself without a common resolution in the abstract and philosophical sense at this time. A government participant, in making the observation of a lack of consensus among the experts, suggested this was "a finding in and of itself." But the importance of the meeting lay primarily in the consciousness-raising about values and ethics in all the participants. It also afforded the opportunity to exchange ideas, discuss issues, cite meaningful experiences, establish new relationships, and, above all, to open communications between different disciplines.

Throughout the workshop discussions, specific references to Dr. Fuchs' and Mrs. Dana's papers were fairly limited. However, the content of the discussion clearly reflected and incorporated the issues raised by both. There was an obvious commitment to struggle with these issues.

When conflict among the group members surfaced, it was lodged in political and philosophical differences, with each adhering to his own previously held beliefs. The confrontation was between philosophical abstractions and pragmatic issues, between health-oriented values and disease-oriented values, between individual actions and group actions. One of the observations made was that the different backgrounds reflecting practice and philosophy revealed interesting and significant gaps in knowledge. It was clear that the philosophers and non-practice professionals were not very familiar with the range and complexity of health care systems nor with alternatives in the organization of health care delivery. In general, there was an undeniable lack of knowledge among the clinicians about administration, social programs, political processes, and broad policy and program demands. There was a split between clinically oriented professionals and policy-planning-oriented professionals. Each was poorly informed about the other and at moments even showed signs of mutual distrust.

The special concerns which entered into group discussions reflected current issues in the society at large. The women's movement, with its challenge to a male-dominated medical system, surfaced in several discussions. The rights and lack of opportunity afforded to minorities arose to dominate one group's discussion. In other groups, physicians dominated, with strongly held commitments to the medical model of care as currently practiced.

All acknowledged the inherent difficulty of value and ethical issues. Also, the field of health planning and health care is so broadly defined as to create a state of confusion about what and how to look at and where to go. The group that dealt with the "aging" seemed to hold their discussion together once they moved away from medical care concerns. Using a defined population and their needs, i.e., the elderly, may have offered more cohesion,

36

particularly evidenced in the group's capacity to address problems in that population and possible plans for solving these problems. It was clear that even when values for health care could be stated, it was very difficult to operationalize them in the total population. Ethics were primarily addressed on a case-by-case basis. Situations were seen as calling for ethical behavior when "good" could be identified in the individual patient, or in the individual provider. One was struck with this case-specific frame of reference to values and ethics without reference to an overall ethical expectation. It seemed that ethical behavior could be spelled out only in the given situation—almost as though "social contract" was encased in spider webs and dusted off only on demand in professional discussions. Another observation was that there was very little discussion of education relating to ethics and values in the professions, except in a sort of apprentice fashion, by attempting to demonstrate ethical behavior in case-by-case situations. The role and responsibility of the educators in relation to value and ethical expectations received very sparse treatment.

Even when there were more questions raised than attempts to answer them, analysis of the spectrum of issues discussed reflected a clustering of thoughts and opinions into several broad areas. These broad perspectives were perceived by the writers as being subdivided as follows:

1. Professionals: Their attitudes and the provider system
2. Consumerism: Patients' rights and responsibilities
3. Consumer and provider issues: Special interest
4. Social choice: The individual and the common good
5. Health planning: Policy making and accountability

The Professionals, and the Provider System

When the working parties considered the health care professionals and the institutional systems in which they practice as a type of special interest group, they concluded that the provider-special interests have determined the way in which health care services are delivered. Opinion prevailed that medicine has influenced the commitments of all other health care professionals, in particular nursing and social work. The institutional programs are those promulgated by academic and clinical medicine and usually are modeled on provider expectations rather than on consumer needs. The assumption under which all have developed their service criteria

37

is that the medical and institutional interests are in the best interests of the patient.

There is no question that the professions bring a special knowledge to health care and that it is this knowledge which gives them the right to perform services. A professional has been socialized into a concept of "social contract." In return for privileges assigned to him by the public, he makes a commitment to public trust and to the public good. However, the interpretation of these tenets is left to subjective determination on both sides and individual biases contribute to the conflict which exists between providers and consumers. Professionals increasingly see themselves as experts in a "speciality," become loyal to that specialty, and want to perform in that perception of their role. For medicine, the training has been for a role in diagnosis and treatment with a commitment to "cure" and the prolongation of life. On the other hand, today's social health care demands are beyond those of illness specificity and related professional specificity. They take us into a complex bio-psycho-social program of care and provision warranting new expertise and awareness about the person, the family, the neighborhood, the environment, and more.

There was consensus among most participants that newly emerging health care professions and paraprofessions are not being given roles and responsibilities that are consistent with a social health care model. It was stated that to achieve such knowledge, it will be necessary to separate and define the role and responsibility of medicine. The old medical model (both in the organization of care and in the education for the profession) is not consistent with the many expectations and changes needed in today's medical care system. The new knowledge, technology, the expectations, and the demands have left everyone unprepared.

The public's long-established view of the physician is one of reverence. However, this attitude has been undergoing change. The questions that the public has raised regarding its health status and the way health care is organized have negatively affected the image of physicians as a group.

The public has not denied the doctor his expert role, but has called for its own role in policy and planning since the public is reluctant to continue with the traditional biases of medicine. The reaction of doctors to these pressures for change has been resistance.

Physicians are more comfortable with individual contracts with their "patients," in the doctor-patient sense, than in addressing the broad social health spectrum. Indeed, most practicing physicians take pride in dealing with individuals on a one-to-one basis. Historically, the physician is trained to reduce pain and suffering and to prolong life expectancy for the individual as well as to eliminate disease. His or her values are those of saving life, reducing disability and suffering, and conquering disease.

When the question was raised as to whether the future medical practitioner in his present student status could be sensitized to the public's expectations, it was doubted that this could be achieved. The reasons cited varied:

1. The vast extent of scientific knowledge that the student must master for basic responsibilities of treatment makes it impossible for him to also be prepared in prevention and social health maintenance.
2. The new objectives cannot be included and thus achieved as long as the educators are themselves the product of the old medical education model.
3. Resistance to change and its anticipated consequences must be expected. Also the present funding patterns support the continuation of the old model.
4. The threat of newly emerging professions and new roles and autonomy for a number of the non-medical health care professionals (e.g., social workers, nursing, midwives) is regarded as entering the area of medical competence, and, for whatever reasons, as undesirable competition.
5. The locus of private practice as solo or group practice limited to doctors only furthers the monolithic approach to service.

The physician, in good faith, sees the medical model in which he practices as an appropriate application of knowledge. The art of listening and interpretation is the creative component of medicine; the "good" physician is seen as one who is able to listen to his patient, obtain "soft" data, and translate this, plus objective findings, into sound diagnosis and a projection of sound treatment for the individual patient. There has been little medical education in the "common good," except for specialists in public health or in community medicine. How to reconcile effectively the individual practitioner's knowledge and skills with those of the community medicine specialist in the public interest is still an open question in this country. There were those in the workshops who suggested that it may be too much to expect the individual who is a surgical expert to be equally expert and responsive in other roles but there are those who suggest that professionals as a group may be able to do so.

From the discussions it was evident that both the social and nursing professions are seen as entrenched alongside medicine. Furthermore, the public sees each as practicing within biases and traditions similar to those of the physicians. They are perceived in their ancillary relationship to doctors, rather than in the new roles which are emerging as a result of new demands and expectations. These professions are in themselves attempting to break from traditional medical care. Social workers have from their beginning carried the special responsibility for mediating between the individual and society's systems of service. It was stated that the problems induced by external factors and internal responses have been the purview of this field. It has carried the dual roles of dealing with social actions for change to affect the external causes and of dealing with the individual in order to cope with his situation in the best way possible. Some noted that the nurse has traditionally met medical expectations by translating them into nursing functions. Both professions have been essentially trapped within the hospital as an organization and have had difficulty in advocating new roles in the total system on behalf of patients' and population needs.

The relationships among professions within health institutions are seen as hierarchical rather than collegial or collaborative in the full sense. The existing team model, so long espoused by all the professions, is not one of equity in partnership, but rather hierarchical, with the doctor claiming the leadership role. The funding for patients' hospital and custodial care in this country is under the jurisdiction of the medical profession.

The institutions are viewed as operating in self-serving ways with a concern for their own survival. Under the circumstances, patients' rights have to contend with provider interests and thus have little chance for realization. Boards of trustees of medical establishments are regarded as representatives of a select segment of the population and tend to be supportive of medicine in its current practices. The general population, as patients, cannot really expect that their rights will be honored until hospitals are accountable to them, until they have representation on the boards. The government has introduced another effort to secure lay involvement in the medical establishment through the enactment of legislation creating the Health Services Administration, with the intent to bring about community participation in local health and hospital affairs.

40

The search is for ways to eliminate the institutional barriers which exclude individuals from care; to find ways for institutions to "listen" to their patients, and to respond to the expressed needs of their own communities. One of the common recognitions which appeared in all groups was that an expert is an "expert" in only one area and does not necessarily carry that status into all other areas. In any case, when an expert and an institution serve as providers they must be accountable not only to the profession or to the institution but to the public they serve. Another opinion repeatedly suggested by the participants was that the mystique of medicine holds dominant in medical institutions and that new movements are resisted in most of those traditional enclaves.

Both the public and physicians have been very slow to respond to prevention as a social health responsibility. The public is slow because it has little knowledge of its potential and because different groups reflect different vested interests; e.g., industrial waste (jobs) and water pollution (drinking and health). Reference was made to women's health groups which have recently sprung up, and to the fact that those supporting midwifery are under legal and professional attack from doctors who wish to close them down, in spite of women's support of their broader prenatal services. The medical establishment has been undermining other professional or special interest groups in their attempts to broaden and organize the delivery of health care, in which doctoring is only one component of a comprehensive service program. The medical establishment is reluctant to relinquish its leadership in the health care field.

The question arises as to whether the public will want and is prepared to wait for medical endorsement of multi-track social health care systems. The reasons cited for social work and nursing readiness is that their education and professional socialization is to the individual client and his social and psychological needs as well as to his medical needs. Physicians' orientation is to scientific knowledge with reference to biologic and clinical concerns in dealing with the human being's illness or disability. When one examines programs serving individuals in hospitals, one sees the frequent absence of social human resources, despite the observed facts that patients present social-psychological concerns that affect their progress. Even administrators of hospitals very often join physicians in their unwillingness to broaden inpatient services to include more comprehensive care.

There was a mixed reaction as to whether new roles for existing

41

professions would indeed produce better programs than those currently under hospital and medical aegis. The concern was that while medical leadership can be evaluated based on data already available, there is no comparable data available to predict the validity of separating nursing and social work with sanctioned autonomy, albeit with accountability. Several participants suggested that the support for separation was present in the historical role of social workers in settlement houses, for example; and that some social work audit data are available even in medical institutions, but have not been made publicly known. It was suggested that the medical profession can accept a team concept of practice wherein the doctor retains final authority and control, but not one of autonomy in others; for this reason, physicians resist social work accountability. It was noted that funding to support studies to demonstrate whether such programs under nursing or social work leadership can be successful is not readily available because allocation of grants is awarded essentially to traditional establishments. There were those in the group who questioned whether social workers and nurses were not in themselves loath to challenge the medical profession openly.

Interestingly, when ethical behaviors in the health care professions arose for discussion, it was the philosophers who offered generalized explanations for what was happening. Ethical principles are under challenge. Too often, professionals operate from a situational demand, exercising ethics to the care and then relating to the consequences rather than to ethical principles. The philosophers referred to this as situational ethics. Ethics are the operational behaviors of values. The observation was made that professionals frequently compromise on behalf of others, but hold to special claims for themselves. It is interesting to note that the systems professionals create for others are not necessarily those they select for themselves when in need. In one group, a quick poll of participants' preferences and usages of health services revealed that all were involved with an individual doctor in private practice. No one used clinics or emergency rooms, although some indicated they would use the latter in the event of a crisis. Professionals do perceive different models of care for those in different socioeconomic classes.

It was agreed that the concept of and expectation in "social contract" was subject to many constraints. The marketplace of services rather than professions' codes of ethics was viewed as the dominant factor in ethical behavior. Economic gain, however, was not seen as the major motivating factor in the breakdown in ethics. The locus of practice, e.g., medical school based hospitals, affects commitments as well. Doctors in these institutions are not rewarded in the same way for providing quality of care as they are for research and concomitant publications. Teaching hospitals, with their educational and research emphases, have values and ethics which can be in conflict with those of the service organizations. Even the rewards in these teaching institutions are the clinical faculty ranks for service and the academic faculty ranks for education and research. The latter are more sought after than the former. When the philosophers viewed ethical behavior, they identified three systems which dictate ethical actions:

1. a system of policed honesty in which the profession's ethics are monitored from within the profession;
2. a system of subjective values which govern our behaviors based on professional socialization of values in the student;
3. a system of universal principles (either God or religiously based or morally-culturally based in values relevant to humanness).

There was a group of non-medical practitioners who suggested that all ethical behavior was currently contaminated by what the members identified as four "devils:" (1) economics, (2) politics, (3) the establishment-system, and (4) more recently, computers. This group felt that the internalization as well as the monitoring of behavior relevant to values had to be incorporated into practice and education.

Consumerism, Patients' Rights and Responsibilities

The issue of consumerism in a service society was raised in almost all the workshops. It was raised in the context of the value "a consumer, an individual has a right to health—and certainly health care." It was recognized that the dilemma has been that few people have addressed the needs of consumers and the special role they should have in services until the advent of Naderism. In a pluralistic society such as ours, the multiple systems of care are ostensibly in competition with each other and are assumed to provide the consumer with choice. But the consumer does not set the rules in these systems of care, and has little input into the means of developing, governing, and delivering care. The priorities and the programs have been set by providers. As we become a more

43

consumer-oriented society, the view has arisen that the consumer has a right to share in the determination of the needs and in shaping the nature of the delivery of services. There are many reactions to consumerism in this form. A number of physicians have resented the interference and wish to return to "status-quoism." There are others who concede that "If consumerism is the price we have to pay, let's get on with it."

The groups recognized that there are different levels of health and different health needs among the various populations of the country. In addition, the nature of available care varies for the different socioeconomic classes. Given the projections in the media of what is available to the public from modern medical technology, expectations are raised and there is a growing public demand for better quality of services. The consumer does not dream of "pie in the sky" in terms of health care. It is the providers who tell him to expect more and who develop the consumer's constantly expanding expectations. The consumer has all the rights of citizenship and in that context has the right to place his demand in the political marketplace.

The interface of diverse opinions regarding the roles and rights of consumers proved to be a discussion heavily charged emotionally. Several participants, speaking for minorities, i.e., those socially and economically disadvantaged and racially discriminated against, viewed our present health care systems as abusive. The position held was that consumerism must be explicit if sound values are to be integrated into care. This means that the recipients of service must have a part in the identification of need and in the decision-making process. Being a part of decision making could enhance the assumption of responsibility in relation to the care received. Blaming the recipient of services for not assuming responsibility for his own health maintenance is a common attitude of providers. In the name of personal self-help, providers neglected to recognize self-help in the governance and organization of services. In addition, opportunity, health education, resources were all too frequently limited and unavailable, particularly to the disadvantaged. Mrs. Dana had cited the danger of further victimizing the victim by holding him to unrealizable expectations in the name of self-help.

Although consumer participation is mandated in some governmental regulations as a value publicly and currently held, it was suggested that providers have granted this only in a pro forma sense and have not truly supported consumer participation. While providers speak to the theory of social justice, they in fact maintain the status quo. The consumer needs to play an active role in the use of the political arena to achieve sound health care services. For this role, the consumer will need to be well-informed. This presents not only problems, but raises questions about his ability to understand and analyze information in an unbiased way. To be informed, the consumer needs to comprehend the differences in attitudes and in expectations among the different peoples in a heterogeneous society.

To understand that suffering may have a religious value to some groups cannot be interfered with, and may influence a person's decision regarding signing a "right to die" request; others will wish to prolong life regardless of the human condition. Another side of the coin is the problem of industrial pollution of drinking waters and the possibility of cancer to the local population in twenty years, and the public's struggle with the choice of its own future public health and its present employment status. In addressing the issue of sound consumerism, there was concern expressed regarding the mobilization of the public without raising excess fear and then precipitating inappropriate individual reaction. There is the factor of the individual's wish for different and new resources to meet his perception of his needs and rights. To be thoroughly informed, the consumer also needs to know how health resources can be reorganized and how he can participate in that reorganization. The lag between what can be ideally planned and its realization is a factor in ongoing conflict when dealing with change.

It is a fact that the acknowledged rights of health care consumers have increased. But rights are complex and difficult to uphold as a constant. The question was raised as to whether "rights" imply benefit to the consumer in all instances. An example of the complexity in health care rights is the one of "informed consent" to procedures and care. The legal profession has been active in pursuing this right for patients. Yet the Karen Quinlan case reflects the degree of conflict that can emerge when "rights" are perceived by different viewers. Another side of the coin was raised with the question "Can the consumer in need of a renal dialysis service be expected to accept that costs for such a program permitting access to all in need may be too much when other health needs are introduced?" Denial of access when in need is unacceptable. When providers have programs to provide, they hold to the right of their availability regardless of cost and even regardless of decreased utilization (e.g., the excess number of hospital beds against need in this country).

It was recognized that with the rise of a strong consumer lobby, relations will develop among groups in order to influence the policy and planning levels of health care. This means that mutual sharing and participation among consumers will become the appropriate mode of communication and even permit the negotiation of ideas to be dealt with, as a start, at the consumer level.

Consumer-Provider Issues, and Special Interests

Consumer movements alone will not necessarily remove the value and ethical dilemmas in health care delivery, since the providers will maintain their role in planning and operation. Because expectations rooted in strongly held sentiments and traditions are slow to change, consumer-provider clashes are to be anticipated.

Can consumers and providers reconcile their differences with and expectations of each other? There were those who perceived the consumers and the providers as two distinct groups with an adversary relationship. In one of the groups, an attempt was made to conceptualize this conflict by describing the different possible types at a one-to-one level of relationship, as in the doctor-patient relationship model:

A.　Some health problems require that the provider be active and the consumer be passive-dependent. Coma is an example. The analogue offered is that of a parent-very young child relationship. Health care professionals are well trained in this mode and adept at dealing in situations which they can control.

B.　Other health problems require that the consumer take some responsibility for his care. The provider must guide, but the consumer must cooperate, assume responsibilities, if the goal is to be achieved. Postoperative convalescence is an example. The analogue cited is the one of parent-adolescent relationship. This is the one in which the health professional attempts to retain control of the relationship, although to a lesser extent than in situation A.

C.　In today's world, most problems in health care require a mutual sharing and participation, calling for rights and responsibilities, between provider and consumer. Chronic illness is an example where participation between client and physician is necessary. The analogue is perceived as adult-to-adult relationship. Yet, because of such factors as socialization and bureaucratization,

46

and of sociocultural and psychological factors as well, mutual participation may be difficult to achieve. It is at this level that health care professionals have the most difficulty and that clients do not know or have difficulty in responding to what is required of them.

It is known that providers will not protect the interests of consumers unless mandated by reimbursing sources. Consumers and providers are distinct and separate groups, each with its own expectations and rule-governed behaviors. An adversary relationship in the general sense, not in the individual caring sense, has inevitably grown up between them.

In considering values, the responsibility is on both consumers and providers to achieve the desirable social health care goal. But are there different values held by each? There is no question that the climate is one of serious difference. Even as the professionals in the workshops moved from the provider to consumer role for themselves, their expectations and demands changed as they shifted positions; the interface of diverse opinions regarding the rights, roles, and responsibilities of consumers and those of professionals and the institutions in which they serve is one which is very heavily charged emotionally, with little expectation for early resolution. It is apparent when one tries to conceptualize the problems or issues for each group that we are not dealing with a unitary set of problems. These concerns may be reflected in disaffection with each other, but that disaffection arises from different expectations and a lack of fulfillment that each has had from the other. One example offered was the recent experience the public had with the swine flu shots, when medical uncertainty and medical politics left the major portion of the public with serious doubts as to the integrity of the recommendation. The aftermath of the flu experience only served to support the public's earlier doubt. This type of illustration was repeated very frequently throughout the day—an overriding example was the media disclosure of the extent of unnecessary surgery performed by ill-equipped professionals.

The observation was made that one of the critical consumer-provider issues was that of "uncertainty." The medical profession is trained never to acknowledge uncertainty. Yet it is the degree to which uncertainty exists as an outcome of care that contributes to consumer disaffection with health providers. The public seeks absolute assurance that medicine in most instances is unable to give. The participants made the observation that where an "outcome" is

47

predictable, it is expert-based and accepted; where the "outcome" is uncertain, then negotiation or conflict between consumers and experts results. Compounding the issue is that the current "caring" system, at least on the institutional level, does not call for self-reliance, but for consumer dependency. When physicians expect self-motivation under some circumstances and dependency in other instances, patients find themselves confused by the conflict in expectations. Moreover all doctors are taught to value "cure" and thus their patients expect it as well. The fact of the matter is that "cure" is impossible in those chronic illnesses which afflict the majority of our population and that individual efforts to prevent diseases are more effective than physicians' care once chronic illness strikes. In the latter instance, all agree that the biggest failure in health care is in our health education programs. Consumers are barraged by a range of educational messages about health care choices, such as the effects of smoking, air and water pollution, overeating, speeding, similar admonitions. The messages treat people as an undifferentiated mass, although in most professional education not only is individual difference taught, but group and familial differences as well. Differences among cultural groups, special interests, and the problems call for different educational approaches.

Special interest groups were seen as a positive factor in that their claims make for diversity in programming. Such groups are consistent, are highly motivated, and act in their own interests. Special interests in the health area include: the unions with the power to lobby; private industry in its practices; the state, through delegated representatives which can establish procedures and policies which in fact regulate the practice; the health care providers, including AHA, AMA and the dozens of professional societies; consumer groups; disease-specific groups; and politicians. Coalition is a frequent maneuver among special interest groups. Politicians move in and out of different coalitions. The reactions of members in the different groups centered more around politicians than any other vested interest. When the political process was raised in terms of health care issues, the groups expressed divergent opinions, reflecting the differences between the practitioners and the planners. There were those who called for the exclusion of the politicians because their input will pollute the "purity" of the proposals. Politicians were seen by clinicians as a special interest group. Some professionals fear even temporary identification with certain political groups; their biases were called to their attention by others. In several of the groups there were those who would include politicians even with eventual compromise to be expected, because in the long run the coalition would permit approval. By including the policy makers in the planning stage, those members believed it was also likely that the policy makers could be held responsible to seek out accountability.

One needs to look at the array of political choices which emerge as a result of multiple interests and expectations. Health has different meanings to different groups. As a concept, health is used to accomplish political purposes. Special interest groups can be very powerful in the policy-making arena (DeBakey and cardiac support; Cooley in relation to anemia; and lay groups for muscular dystrophy, renal disease, et al.).

It is agreed that while people can respond to information when it is meaningful to them, information alone will not change behavior. The creation of sound and effective health education measures will require considerably more attention on the part of providers and more understanding by consumers of ways to make concerns meaningful enough to act in one's own self-interests.

To deal with patients' rights and responsibilities requires an active program of interpretation. It is not enough to develop a patients' rights pamphlet for circulation among users; in addition, the provider and the consumer must assist each other in developing responsibilities for interpretation. Patients' rights need to be known by patients, but they must also be soundly interpreted to those who provide services. When both consumers and providers are seen as having rights and responsibilities, then perhaps a partnership can come about.

Most participants agree that effective care requires a redistribution of power from the "experts," to share between the provider and the consumer. While the expert has a role, he is no more value-free than the consumer; instead, his values are different from the consumer's. One should not attribute bias-free judgment to the "expert" for anything. One can assign specialized knowledge to the "expert" and draw on that when needed, but one should not assume that personal, subjective, and special interests do not exist. A partnership of mutual participation and mutual benefits can be dealt with openly. Since all professionals tend to impose a degree of dependency on their clients, the prediction is that consumerism will conflict with providerism until such time as consumers are treated as partners in direct service, in assessment of services, in planning, and in policy determination. Consumerism is seen as offering the potential for provider-client relationships characterized by mutual participation. One of the present barriers to this is that professionals believe they have first call on what is "right" and leave little input to the design by the client. The consideration in reaching a working model between consumer groups and provider groups is not exclusion of one or the other from the policy, planning, and implementing stages. The mature adult-to-adult mutual participation model is recommended. Can it be achieved?

Social Choice, the Individual, and the Common Good

When we examine the issues in social choice, there is general recognition that we are dealing with the failure of society to respond to the entire spectrum of human needs. But, as stated by one of the participants, "If you think about the whole too long, you get angry: you must partialize it out." That health systems must stand for the common good was readily agreed upon; the achievement of this goal in the light of limited resources was recognized as the hardship. There was general agreement that the capacity of the health care system to absorb unlimited dollars appears to be overwhelming, and that we must face up to the fact that there is a limit to what we can spend today. It was also recognized that the systems we have today reflect present-day societal values; that this raises all kinds of questions about basic values and complex problems about future fundamental needs and values.

Survival and "dying" were widely discussed value concerns. Who shall survive and the quality of survival was deliberated, using the popularized Karen Quinlan case. The question arises as to whether survival is a value with priority demand on resources ahead of improved social functioning. This conflict recurred over and over again in the discussions. Another critical incidence cited was that of derelicts who, after years of self-abuse, develop kidney malfunction, making them eligible for very expensive renal dialysis treatment, and who are seen as a continuing unproductive drain on society. This clearly demarked the conflict between patients' rights and patients' responsibilities, on the one hand, and the responsibilities of those who provide care, on the other. The value of treating when cure or correction is slim was questioned. Despite these illustrations of the individual versus the common good, the option for personal

50

and personalized choice was never relinquished by most of the participants.

Do individual "rights" emerge now as an issue because of limiting and diminishing resources in the world and in the environment, or because it is difficult to find a balance between better health and overall economic development? Since we have faced one crisis after another, is crisis a catalyst-raising concern over values and ethics similar to those raised as a result of reduced resources? A few were reminded of the Depression of the 1930s when resources were so limited that human survival in terms of food and shelter was translated into social security and work programs as society's primary value. Values and ethics seem of less concern to professions and public alike during periods of great affluence when all needs can have some access to partial resolution. When crisis and diminishing resources are upon us, then competing interests appear to claim their share over others.

Existing human and material resources are not being used to best advantage. One group tried to define the situation out of which problems in the delivery of health care have emerged. Someone with experience in Third World health systems suggested that Fuchs' analysis did not touch upon the realities which define the situation in much of the world today. Fuchs calls for explicit choices reflective of democratic principles. Yet much of the world lives in non-democratic regimes where choices are not made in an open political forum. Nevertheless, it was suggested that in socialistic countries health care usually receives a high priority, whereas in capitalistic systems, health care is granted a low priority. Capitalistic countries need to realize that "Health is an investment which gives a return." The issue was further expanded when discussing the responsibilities to be assumed by consumer and provider in terms of mutual participation. In particular reference to prevention, the issue of individual choice and liberty was raised in terms of society's right to mandate health practices which might clash with individual preferences. Our own society tries to solve this dilemma by providing incentives for valued behavior. At the federal level, incentives take the form of grants to health institutions. At the same time, private control over new communication networks such as TV, newspapers, magazines, and so on can direct resources to those health expenditures that offer financial gains and thus determine what kind of information to disseminate. Because health information in the public interest is not profit-producing, it may not be

51

of interest to the private sector which controls the mass media. Are these the same reasons practicing physicians have not played a role in trying to influence the mass media in relation to health maintenance?

As the issues became more specific, the sources of conflict were made more apparent. This occurred in one of the discussion groups when public health needs and societal needs were juxtaposed against industry's needs. The recent controversy over asbestos was seen to illustrate a critical dilemma in social health planning involving what may be viewed as a discrepancy between the goals of private enterprise and the goals of health and illness prevention. The asbestos industry withheld information that the so-called "Zero-Dust Solution," which would have significantly reduced the health hazard from airborne asbestos dust particles, was feasible. Instead, the industry argued that to interfere in any way with its current mode of production would result in economic destruction of the industry with a significant loss of jobs to the national economy. The threat of increased unemployment made politicians wary of placing controls on the production of asbestos, even though present methods were clearly a health hazard. The political process was impeded in its search for a solution to a major health problem because the industry—out of a motive for optimal profit—withheld important information. Investigation further revealed that physicians employed by the asbestos industry did not properly refer patients who had contracted diseases caused by exposure to asbestos. Consequently, while the patients were treated for their disease, the public remained unaware of the magnitude of the health threat posed by asbestos. This, of course, raises another social health dilemma: that of the values which guide the health professional who works within the private market mechanism. Do professionals in bureaucracies tend to be transformed in such a way that the universalistic and humanitarian values assumed to be part of the professional ethic become replaced by pragmatic, corporation-oriented values?

A counterbalance to the power of private industry is the labor union. In the asbestos case, the unions were in the forefront of the move to protect people from this health hazard. Nevertheless, it was generally agreed among the participants that unions, as well as private industry, have narrowly defined goals and biases which do not take the larger social good into account. This is again the issue of how much freedom a free society can allow.

Access and increasing access to health and medical care seem to be a prime value. Health systems need to be opened up to give the public as much as it has the right to expect. But as we increase access, and our systems of care grow bigger, does depersonalization result, with a decline in individualization?

However, when access is examined by practitioners, they see that it is dictated by the time and resources that are allocated. We need to assess the problems that arise because consumer needs are not always compatible with the current framework for service delivery. It was recognized that if we wish to guarantee access, then choice may have to be eliminated. This would then jeopardize other values we hold. There are competing values in relation to access. Some are:

a. to each according to his needs;
b. to each according to what he produces;
c. to the segment of society;
d. to the whole of society.

It is suggested the systems of care reflect the values currently held, or those held in the immediate past.

While there is always the need to look at broader societal issues, no one is willing to relinquish individual choice.

The questions arise over and over again of discrepancies between individual needs and the needs of society, the definition and the resolution of those needs. The existence of discrepancies suggests that our big challenge is to bring about reallocation of resources. All believe that choices can be made today which were not possible in earlier times. New technology can be an asset, but sometimes it can override individual choice.

Some value stances can be in conflict with other values. Even if general values were agreed upon, there remain individual, personal values that influence delivery of services at the practitioner level. We need to look at the professional's enactment of values as well as values at the abstract level. All members in all of the groups agreed that ethical principles and values must come into play in order to make choices (yet the groups had trouble identifying which were primary). It is clear to most that economic conditions may be the vehicle forcing us to choose among values. But just because we can and do make choices does not mean we have settled the values issues. When a problem is germane to a specific segment of society its value is viewed as primary by that group which presses for legislation in its interest. However, the question was raised as to whether professional values can shift and change with each special interest group's pressure. While equity and an egalitarian thrust need to be considered, the application of professional knowledge must nevertheless take precedence. This is perceived as the essence of professionalism. Professions carry social responsibility inherent in their training and in their knowledge. Moreover the professions have assumed and been granted leadership roles by the public in return for commitment to the public good. This is the social contract which should be institutionalized into professional behavior.

Different disciplines have different approaches to social choice. It is speculated that many of the service professions' codes are profession-related rather than in the public good.

Social Workers: addressed social choice in terms of health in the broad spectrum of social need with their perception of impact on physical and mental health, drawing on social justice and equity of access.

Hospital Administrators: expressed responsibility in social choice as providing the best care, to the greatest number in the best possible ways, within the resources available.

Philosophers: perceived social choice in a framework of social contract with its rights, obligations, duties, roles, space agreements, social organization. The questions they raised dealt with an organic view of society and in what way we are a part of each other.

Physicians: held to their commitment (1) to reduce suffering; (2) to prevent or eliminate disease, and (3) to prolong life. They have been trained to curative medicine in a biomedical mold. The commitment is the application of knowledge in the treatment of the individual.

In contrast, physicians trained in

Community Medicine: made explicit their values by expressing the belief that the community has a right to determine its priorities and to identify the health care it wishes to become involved with. A shared interrelationship between local consumers and local providers was advocated.

The social choices restated: "Is health care a right? If health is a right, which is it?" Each makes for different demands on and expectations of the professionals, of the consumers as individuals, and of society in general.

Health Planning, Policy Making, and Accountability

In a pluralistic society, the differential needs and demands of different groups are always a problem. Whether in times of affluence or in limitation, planning is required. At this time, when the nation has become conscious about the shortage of resources, we have no other choice but to engage in planning based on the clear notion that resources are inevitably limited.

There was a recognition and concern that the national perspective in planning for health services is disconnected from ethical considerations. Current health programs are not designed to provide better health. At present, health planning efforts are too often based on provider needs, rather than on population needs. Physicians and the instruments of service, referred to as the medical model, determine what care to give and how it can be given. Current health care programs are in general limited to the medical care of disease and disability. It is essentially a "sick" care system. Given consumer needs and present health and health care resources, the two must be brought closer together through meaningful social planning. But the questions rose again and again with limited answers:

> How do you meet population needs and expectations within limits of resources or organization? How do you deal with patient expectation in the face of limited resources? How do you deal with provider needs in light of population needs?

Given the state of deficits in our knowledge, and the complexity of the issues, who should do the planning? Participants in general agreed that one cannot rely exclusively on the "experts" for overall determinations. Furthermore, they felt that at least two broad categories of experts, the planners and the doers (the professional providers), still need to learn how to work together. These experts should be involved in the marketplace of ideas and as consultants while the political process should be left to the final "arbiters." Someone said it in this way: "The technicians should be on 'tap' not on 'top'." The policies are separate from the planning process. Planning is influenced by the biases and values held by the planners. Planning and policy call for a healthy relationship between consumers and providers, allowing for negotiation and compromise. And given the same deficit in our knowledge, how shall we do the hard planning? Must we not start by identifying the problems and establishing priorities among them? Everyone felt concern about organizational problems in health care services, the inequity of access and availability, the issue of quality and accountability, the lack of systems of care; financial arrangements and misutilization of resources were strongly debated.

Problems of choice were, of course, discussed. There was also concern that the national perspective in planning for health services is disconnected from ethical expectations and that no cohesive value base exists in dealing with health care. This may be seen in the fragmentation in systems of delivery, in the lack of relationship between needs and resources, and in that means and ends seem so little connected. When the medical establishment alone identifies health problems, it tends to perceive them in terms of epidemiology, prevalence, morbidity, mortality, treatment, cure as in biomedical or in public health concepts. Everyone acknowledged the validity of such dimensions, but many voices also addressed the broader perspectives involving social-psychological and cultural claims on the planning process. All the groups called for the participation of different professions and of consumers in the identification of problems and their priorities. In setting priorities, it was fully recognized that the one big problem is finding *consensus*. The discussion revealed that there is little in the way of a consensus model in today's planning. Instead, it has been replaced by a *conflict* model. This takes note of the formation of coalitions among different interest groups, each with its priorities and strategies for achieving its ends. The consumer movement can create powerful interest groups from the client sector and can bring other sectors into coalition. The providers create their coalition, too. However, in the short run at least, planning can be even more complex because coalitions tend to change their membership as the task at hand changes. Any planning system must bear in mind the natural resistance to change in individuals and institutions.

Planning was ideally viewed by many as an ongoing process that involved the definition of objectives based on priority needs, the reorganization of resources as a method to meet those objectives, and evaluation activities that would lead to the redefinition of goals and objectives. If defining priorities was viewed as difficult, reaching consensus in objectives was viewed as even more difficult. Attempts were made to identify some objectives for a social health care system as advocated by Mrs. Dana. A pluralistic approach offering choice but safeguarding opportunity to comprehensive care was seen as compatible with American expectations. Such care could also have its locus in any system of services, even outside the traditional medical establishment. The interdependence of systems was viewed as a meaningful way to deal with needs and resources. A revision of the reward system to professionals was considered to be necessary. In terms of resources reorganization, one of the current attempts to reorder the delivery of care system was illustrated, that of separating hospital care and ambulatory care services. When such separation was discussed, the hospitals were regarded as under the purview of physicians and hospital administrators, while ambulatory care was perceived as the social health system under the direction of a mix of professionals from different health disciplines with a more comprehensive orientation to service. In evaluation, full recognition was given to the fact that periodic documentation is needed to measure the effectiveness as well as the efficiency of the programs. Health planners have to lay out social indicators and convert them into measurable objectives. All agreed that clarity of function in relation to goals needs to be objectified in accountability terms, but current attempts to make the health delivery system accountable to society are limited, and the evaluation component of resource allocations is still in the dark ages. Medical audit systems are currently operating at beginning levels and on problems which are not specific indicators of the quality of health, but rather on the effectiveness of the delivery of care of the given institutions.

As much as values are necessary for decision making, so is technical knowledge. We tend not to evaluate what we are doing but continue to spend money. We need evaluations, data for decision making. Most policy is not rational and is based on incomplete information. It may be rational in terms of moving from here to there, but we have to ask if the end product is rational. So health policy planning proceeds without sufficient data, with poor evaluative tools, without the skills base for making high-level decisions, and with a shortage of policy makers. Some of the key questions requiring answers that would affect the way health care is delivered are: "Why do people use health services?" "Do existing health care systems create needs and their own continued existence?" "What range of manpower is needed?" "Can physician-extenders be used effectively?" "How can we expand the role of the MD so that his time and skills are used most effectively?" Unless answers to questions such as these are forthcoming, planning and distribution of health resources will continue to be on a hit-or-miss basis.

A health planning process requires us to keep in mind not only what *should* be done, but what is actually do-able. Ethical choices are not incompatible with the need for rational planning since planning itself is influenced by the value systems of the planners. Most policy and planning programs have no macro-system staff trained for high-level functioning. Planning in terms of the problems we are wrestling with needs a healthy relationship between provider and consumer. Planning is more realistic and has a better chance of working when those who implement it are involved in the planning process.

The planning process is regarded as a dynamic one that should lead to change involving the planner, the doer, and the consumer. These three are not one-on-one, but are instead interactional. However, we must recognize that limited knowledge is a fact of life to be built into and coped with in the planning process.

Policy Making

How to influence policy and change the system was viewed as the crucial issue. How to establish priorities, who makes decisions, and who should make them was considered the crux of the health care system dilemma. The dilemma imposed is that society wants one standard of care, yet the distribution and allocation of resources are in conflict with that standard. The differing demands of different interests lead to political conflict and then to political resolution. There is no agreement as to whether there is enough or too little in the health care system. Participants claim the need to look at all parts of the system and not just one (e.g., hospitals). In any case, diversification and pluralism were supported by most of the participants, although it was recognized that another type of socialized order than the one we live in could produce a monolithic and perhaps more efficient health maintenance system.

If we wish to contemplate change in the delivery of care, then we need to face the structure and the problems inherent in *change*, which inevitably lead to political constraints. In all change, broader political issues are at stake than those that appear on the surface. One of the participants said "What capitalistic countries need to realize is that health is an investment which gives a return." Some socialistic countries have achieved certain health goals not achieved in the United States. This is illustrated by our relatively unfavorable life expectancy and infant mortality rates. Does the political and economic system serve as a deterrent to rational policy making? There are many factors which prevail against social change. Institutional structures and personnel with their established programs make it very difficult to obtain organizational shifts.

One issue that will need to be addressed by policy makers and the public is whether the attitudes and behavior so frequently seen in profit-making industry are also being evidenced in the so-called socially oriented health care industry. The question arises as to whether the health care industry is under the control of a well-placed power elite whose interests are self-serving rather than directed to the public good. The participants noted the significance of power groups in our society and the impact of some of them on health care programming. All of the working parties held that quality of care must be available to all segments of society with no concentration on either the well-to-do or the disadvantaged. The needs of all would somehow have to be met equitably. This followed on one group's contention that certain minorities had been disenfranchised from good care and that special corrective measures were obligatory.

When the groups examined who are the parties involved in decision making in health, they ranged the gamut from professionals, to consumers, to politicians, and on. They were concerned that university-based health care professionals monopolize the means of analysis of health care programs, thus controlling assessment and prediction. Their institutional biases, whether in the role of teacher or provider, were cited. Some saw professionals in the role of technical expert, thus influencing policy making. All the groups agreed with Dr. Fuchs that professionals should serve in advisory and not in decision-making capacities with reference to policy determination. It was felt that non-health care professionals, i.e., laypersons, can be better entrusted to reach final policy decisions. The Congress, representing its constituencies, is more apt in the final analysis to be responsive to public than to provider needs. Thus people, through their representatives, are seen as in a position to set policy. However, all agreed that policy processes do need to be brought into proximity with the programming processes.

It was recognized that unless those making the decisions are different from the do-ers, there is no assurance that any change can occur. Access into and participation in the process (all these participants "wanted in") does not necessarily change the outcome (but could change the goals), yet it does heighten the investment of special interests and brings in different viewpoints. Some suggested that perhaps a "sunshine" expectation in health care policy making would be desirable.

When resources are limited, who should have the priorities? All alternatives have serious potential difficulties. Decisions are too frequently made on the basis of costs rather than on need and value of a service. One of the philosophers suggested that sometimes no one wanted to assume responsibility for an answer. He posited a set of alternatives:

> those with seniority
> those who did the most for society
> a random basis.

In all, it was agreed that none of these alternatives would or should survive a decision-making process.

If we had unlimited resources would the policy-making process be different? The issues to be faced are probably the same, but the resolution process may be less complicated. Some suggested that affluence may create more struggles in relation to decision making. Others suggested that more caring services would arise and perhaps more ideas would be projected as resolutions. The problems of assessment in determining valid choice and in planning for the next steps would be the same under affluent or limited resource availability. It is believed that under any set of circumstances no program can be designed that would not disadvantage some group.

One of the workshop groups projected alternative policies for the availability and organization of health care in this country. A rationale for each was developed.

Health Care System I

    a.   Program: A National Health System (Universal)
1. no free choice
2. no private, fee-for-service care
3. all health care free and readily available
4. health education free and a component of the system
5. organized in a health center (not hospital-based) for a given geographic population. The staffing is multidisciplinary to include: internist, pediatrician, public health

60

nurse, social worker, family health worker. The center would serve hospitals and nursing homes in the region.
  6. entitlement to all components of the program would be based on citizenship.
  b. Rationale; to guarantee equal access to all, better distribution on geographic and local area basis, and better utilization of manpower and resources.

Health Care System II

  a. Program: National Health Insurance (Universal)
    1. provision of pluralistic choice in health care; e.g., HMO or fee-for-service
    2. choice of physician
    3. back-up services of regional hospital for all systems under *I*
    4. regional emergency services available to all in need
    5. health education available within the system of care selected.
  b. Rationale: The same as in *I*, but suggests comprehensive care can be given without the state control of all institutions.

There was some discussion regarding experience to date with prepaid group practice plans. There was evidence of some concern with organizational problems in such programs as HIP. On the other hand, the Kaiser-Permanente and Puget Sound experiences were offered as demonstrating that similar shared goals by consumers and providers can result in a sound program, and built-in checks and balances to safeguard both consumer and provider interests.

A critical policy issue in relation to payment to the provider of care received special attention. There was recognition of the multiple sources which have made a major stronghold of a fee-for-service system. The dynamic of that pressure group is to perpetuate "fee-for-service." However, there will need to be acknowledgement very soon that forty percent (40%) of medical care costs derive from the public dollar, and a substantial percentage is represented in insurance coverage on behalf of the public. These sources have some claim in determining the payment method. There are supports for maintaining a "fee-for-service" method in that it is perceived as having a value of control for the provider. There are those who see

61

in capitation the value of control for the consumer. Others challenge the actuality of both of these statements, reflecting that lack of opportunity, lack of access, and lack of knowledge are prime impediments to freedom of choice.

One of the conclusions for policy which arose is that minimal standards for health maintenance will need to be achieved. This is more than medical care. It was suggested that in the future dollars going into medical care will need to be diverted into social health care programs.

Helen Rehr, D.S.W.
Director, Department of Social Work Services
The Mount Sinai Hospital
Edith J. Baerwald Professor of Community Medicine (Social Work)
Mount Sinai School of Medicine
City University of New York

Samuel J. Bosch, M.D.
Associate Professor of Community Medicine
Mount Sinai School of Medicine
City University of New York

Values and Ethical Dilemmas in Relation to the Delivery of Socio-Health Care to the Aging[1]

GIDEON HOROWITZ

JOHN P. MAHER

The Special Workshop on the Aged of the Doris Siegel Memorial Colloquium provided its participants with a highly provocative, enriching, and, at the same time, somewhat frustrating experience. This essay represents a digestion and exposition of the content, discussions, minutes, and "sense of meeting" of the all-day workshop, rather than an attempt at reporting the exact feelings, verbatim arguments, agreements, or disputes of the workshop participants; these were aired in the context of a free-wheeling give-and-take, spread out over several hours of repartee between representatives from the fields of sociology, gerontology, medicine, social work, philosophy, and education, each with an interest in and a commitment to the health care of the aged.

The enormity of the workshop agenda was immediately apparent, and sufficiently overwhelming so that the chairman's opening remarks were met with a classical "awkward pause," while the group participants struggled with the impact and intent of value and ethical dilemmas as outlined in the suggested workshop agenda.

The initial silence was ultimately broken by a comment from the sole medical member of the workshop, cautioning the group to be mindful that just as "no man is an island," so too every categorical problem of the aged (whether medical, health, economic, social, political, educational. etc.) ultimately reflects upon all the others; that, in effect, the elderly (like the poor and other underprivileged minorities) find themselves in the center of an intricate network of problems; of an ecology of "health" and "illness," using these terms in their broadest sense.

This notion was immediately seized upon by various participants and served as a springboard for a discussion of the inconsistencies and contradictions in values which our society holds in regard to the aging. It was clear that society does make a series of value judgments regarding the aging, but it was less clear what the total thrust of these values is, how they are determined, and what the various social systems are which impact upon the aging.

Economic Factors

It was suggestd that our society seems to suffer from "value schizophrenia." On the one hand, the aging are only perceived as valuable while they are in the economic system and productive. The young, children and adolescents, are valued because of their economic productive potential; adults up to the age of 65 are certainly regarded as currently economically productive and therefore rate high on this economic materialistic scale. Yet, despite previous contributions and productivity, the aged are considered neither potentially nor currently productive and thus rate very low on such a value scale. On the other hand, American society, at least as indicated through its elected representatives, did put an economic (and therefore a health) value on the aged with the passage of social health legislation (Medicare and Medicaid) in the mid-1960s, and in subsequent legislation aimed specifically at improving the lot of the elderly. A similar "schizophrenia" is seen in some of the available support systems; e.g., the social welfare system has automated SSI to improve the provision of one kind of service to the aged, but has concomitantly lost sight of the individual and his/her particular needs and problems.

There seemed to be consensus that the foregoing statements regarding the low economic valuations of the aged were compatible with certain points made by Dr. Fuchs in his keynote speech, leading to the next obvious question; namely, that if the aged are viewed as being on the bottom of our economic value scale, should not more of society's money and efforts be invested in caring/providing for the younger age groups rather than for the aged?

The members seemed to feel that this was an economic straw man, an artificial way of posing the question. They pointed out that our values, like the aged themselves, were not, and should not be, of one piece—each is composed of different subsets or subgroupings, which historically have tended to change over time and in reaction to extrinsic changes in society, its institutions, and the perceived interrelationships between groups. For example, it was pointed out, the aged are a multifaceted group; furthermore, society is not actually "keeping them alive"; in fact, their longevity and their increasing numbers and proportions are a result of society's efforts and expenditures in keeping children alive. This would almost imply that the *first question* (societal versus individual needs) actually represented a false dichotomy, and that because of the ecology of health, alluded to earlier, all age groups are actually interrelated if not interdependent. Certain members indicated, therefore, that in considering the question of priorities, and the social health needs of people, we were perhaps really addressing the question of *quality of life* at whatever age.

As another example of this interrelationship of subsystems, it was pointed out that "the aging," in addition to having their own problems and needs, can also markedly affect other groups and society as a whole by acting as a political force (witness the Grey Panthers, the voting record of senior citizens, and so on). This exchange prompted references to Dr. Fuchs' caution to "beware the expert" of one field when he (or we) defines and determines overall values, or values in a different field.

Societal Factors

Taking the question of how our society determines its value priorities still further, it was noted that certain other factors may be operational here. (1) Our society tends to give to a group not necessarily in accordance with that group's needs, but in accordance with society's political, social, and economic determinations; and gives just sufficiently to avoid a revolution or a major social/political upheaval; i.e., the squeaky wheel gets just sufficient grease to tone down or barely halt the squeak. When we (society) misjudge, riots, political upheavals, and/or revolutions occur. This may have particular relevance to "the aging," since, as their numbers increase quantitatively, they become potentially more powerful politically and socially. (2) The historical development of American social welfare systems and programs is permeated by a certain "moralistic" tone: we give to people "when it's not their fault;" e.g., the blind, the orphaned, and the disabled veterans; but not to the alcoholics, the drug addicts, or "other criminals" or deviants. This value system is also applicable to the aged, who for many years were active, productive, contributing members of society, and who have now grown old and feeble through no fault of their own.

In the ensuing discussion, the group struggled with conceptualizing the value dilemmas in relation to the delivery of social health care. There was general agreement that the concepts of "need" and "not being at fault" accounted in part for the allocation of services to the aging, despite their resting on the low end of the economic value scale. (3) The guilt feelings of the younger population were another factor cited. Most young people tend to feel that they should be responsible for their parents when the latter grow old and feeble. There is a human relationship involved here, which eventually becomes translated into social legislation such as Medicare. Because of some of these "human" factors, it was pointed out, it would be highly problematic to attempt a rigid economic "costing out" of the "pool of credits" earned during one's economically productive years and relate it to the benefits granted to the aged.

There was a generally negative reaction toward identifying productivity as the sole determinant of value, and the group was especially uncomfortable with using only an economic rationale as the argument in support of programs for the aging. One participant reminded the group that society, through its social legislation, has stated that health itself is not only a value but a right. Furthermore, it was pointed out, we frequently accept the false generalization that the aged are unproductive and largely dependent. It is important to note in this regard that nationally the majority of aged are *not* economically dependent (except, perhaps, upon their own social security payments); that some do remain productive well into the 70s and 80s; and that undoubtedly many more would remain productive, were it not for mandatory retirement regulations and federal disincentives.

Biomedical Factors

From the medical-biologic point of view, most of man's physical faculties seem to peak in his 20s–30s. This seems to be supported by recent work at Stanford University, which indicates that the force of mortality tends to double every eight to ten years after age 30. In such a context, humans could actually be said to start aging at 30 years, and aging itself becomes a logical and necessary step in the progression of growth and development.

It was also noted that, because of our national tradition and economic history, we seem to have an illusion of economic omnipotence: given enough money, we can conquer all our problems and fulfill all our needs. In this context it was pointed out that medicine and society, in a sense, have fed this illusion by "conquering" so many medical-health problems in this century that surely the vision of immortality is almost in sight. We seem to expect that all chronic and debilitating problems can be overcome as were many of the acute and infectious diseases prevalent during the first half of this century; that indeed the process of aging itself can be delayed or indefinitely deferred. What we once sought through magic, we now expect from medicine. We have progressed from the Fountain of Youth to rejuvenation to cryonics and regeneration. Yet, even at the more realistic level of continuing research and treatment of chronic diseases, costs have escalated to such an extent that it may simply be economically impossible to make any meaningful progress in these areas. Similarly, it was predicted, we will see that the major limitation in developing and delivering optimum social services is also the economic factor.

Political Factors

This led some members of the group to the assertion that we had been overlooking a central issue in the discussion thus far; namely, that our political compromises have played a major role in the allocations of limited resources and in allowing providers to limit services; certainly, Medicaid could have been a totally different and progressive process, rather than a political afterthought and un-planned "sleeper."

On this issue of the impact of politics, there was considerable give-and-take, with a somewhat confused exchange of semantic approaches to the various definitions and applications of "politics." Despite the fact that some felt the group was talking in a tangential way and was having trouble in organizing all this, there was agreement that politics was a major factor (related to, but distinct from economics) affecting social health care, and the concern was expressed that we, as professionals, and as "experts" in our respective fields, were not feeding accurate and up-to-date information and data regarding the actual capacities and needs of the aging to the "decision makers," the elected politicians, as well as to society as a whole.

With increasing tempo, the participants struggled to pull together sometimes mutual and sometimes disparate points of view concerning values, value systems, the roles of professionals, and of politicians.

It was emphasized in a variety of ways that decisions are made at many levels, and that whether we called them politicians, legislators, or statesmen, the decision makers in our pluralistic society had to be influenced by a plethora of inputs, data, pressures, and the like. In this kind of system, therefore, it was important to have everyone understand that the economist is only one of many voices, be he staff man or lobbyist for a special interest; we must assume and require that economics be a scientific tool for data-gathering as a *base* for the decision-making process, but that it be only *one* of many such tools which underpin the social health delivery system and which help us to determine what value systems we supply, and whether we are doing so correctly. Furthermore, in such a system, the "professionals" would also be merely one type of expert in the decision making and prioritization of values. In addition to fostering their own values and interests, the professionals would also, it is hoped, act as representatives or ombudsmen for their patients or clientele, and might best play this role as active participants in regional planning for social health care.

In this type of ideal political system, allowing for diverse inputs, evaluations, and decision making, there was one principal ethical issue which was brought up and not really resolved to anyone's satisfaction; i.e., the ethical problem of what appears to be a separation of conscience from the politician. If we are to avoid the extremes of bald economic decision making on the one hand, and of totalitarian arbitrariness on the other, do we not require of our elected representatives that their decisions be tempered with justice, humanity, and the ethical values inherent in our social structure and our common law?

Here, it was suggested that we had been thinking too much in terms of politicians, and perhaps not enough in terms of politics and the political system as it is currently functioning.

Educational Factors

Given their increasing numbers and their growing political clout as mentioned earlier, why cannot a population such as the aged be educated to understand that repressive legislation is not effective or desirable? At this point, reference was made to an earlier exchange dealing with calls for harsh legislation as a response to increased muggings and crimes of violence perpetrated against the elderly. To balance this, educational efforts could be aimed at the aged to enlighten and motivate them in relation to identifying and pushing for their own programs, needs, creative legislation, and so on.

Essentially, the group was saying that our influence as professionals should be exerted simultaneously in two directions—on the politician *and* on the consumer—and that we appear to be projecting a continuum which runs from *needs* to *rights* to *absolute rights*. Yet it was pointed out that in continuing these deliberations we must remember that we, too, are not "value-free" and must avoid the traditional tendency of other experts to dictate a system constructed of our own values and beliefs.

Socio-Ethical Factors

The remainder of the morning session reverberated around a number of questions, problems, areas of uncertainty and/or inadequate data, which can be lumped loosely, for want of a better term under the broader heading of "socio-ethical."

One example of this was the question of whether the real problem of the aging in this context was really age, as such, or whether their problems were not similar and parallel to those of other minorities, underprivileged, and underrepresented subgroups in our overall population. In this case, the effect would be to require a different approach to analyzing the roots of the problem, as well as different approaches to developing solutions to the problem.

From a philosophical point of view, it was suggested that the rights to "life, liberty, and the pursuit of happiness" are accepted and presumably guaranteed in our earliest American political documents. Our latter-day representatives (and a goodly proportion of our population), as well as our professionals, state that these rights require a high quality of health and medical care as a prerequisite or a *sine qua non*. What this resolves itself to, then, is that we have been actively criticizing our system for its deficiencies in terms of (a) the right to care, and (b) equal access to quality care. In the past, society's attitudes on life, death, and health have reflected deep historical, religious, and philosophical convictions. Now we are seeing great modification in earlier value systems. There is now a great deal of respect for the "sanctity of health" as well as of life. Furthermore, it was stressed that the concept of health is not identical with medical care, but is much broader, and that physicians produce only a small, though very important, proportion of total health care.

69

On the other hand, we have a system more and more based on purely economic values: efficiency, productivity, cost-effectiveness. Hospital beds have to be kept filled (Roemer's Law). A vast amount of money is poured into the care of the elderly and chronically ill, with an unknown (but presumably very significant) proportion being paid out for the last ten days to two weeks of life. Much of the care for the elderly is either custodial or crisis-oriented, rather than aimed at prevention and health maintenance.

This points up another very real ethical economic dilemma; namely, that from the standpoint of government and of economics, it may not be "worthwhile" to save an old person's life. If economics is all that counts (and we keep coming back to that issue), then "value" comes out in terms of "cost control." In this type of system, economic judgments have been made by the legislators that, beyond a certain point, costs, and not rights or other values, will be the determining factor; that someone is going to be killed, or at least be allowed to die, because of economic factors. Concurrently, there is an attitudinal, judgmental aspect, which leads almost no one to want to care for the aged: their families reject them; acute care hospitals only want them while they are sick, treatable, and "interesting"; the government is interested in cost controls; and third parties commonly refuse to underwrite preventive and/or ambulatory care.

Health as a "gestalt" encompasses more than just medical and clinical factors. Yet we stand by while our current system continues to fragment or segment man via categorical programs, Medicaid restrictions, or nursing home "predictor scores." Thus, our present system is not framed in terms of people nor of human values. The more complex our society has become, the more we have broken down into segregated, bureaucratic ways of functioning.

Since we implement the overall system, who should be the moralists? How do we become aware of the fact that we are participating in economic decisions which kill, or at least permit people to die—and all this based upon what we consider the wrong values and reasons? These ethical questions cry out for examination! Yet how do we develop a system which can tell us over long periods of time what the ethical and health patterns are; how to get the facts, or know what to do? In effect, our decision *not* to act, *not* to examine, *not* to alter the values and decision-making process, is a decision to accept the status quo; to make the current system work.

70

"Our" Values

Summarizing the process the participants had gone through, the chairman observed that we had analyzed a number of problem areas, and had tentatively tried several potential approaches to developing solutions, but in another sense had reacted by ascribing the problems to a series of "devils": economics, politics, computers, the system, and so on. How then, he asked, are we to deal with what we won't accept? What is *our* role as practitioners and as change agents? Where and what are our own values, especially in relation to the rights of patients, confidentiality, and the like?

In their struggle to respond to these points, the participants recognized that in our society (unlike, say, the Orient) age itself has a negative value, irrespective of health, with each generation increasingly rejecting the elderly (nuclear versus extended family; institutionalization of the aged): the ultimate rejection becomes euthanasia. While no one was sure how society reached this point, it was clear that our individual philosophies and value systems guide us in what we do. Our own values are expressed in our work, in the positions we take.

By consensus, the members agreed that all people have a right to health care. In the particular case of the aged, we are dealing with a population we have never had before, in terms of longevity, numbers, education, and influence. Moreover, "the aging" are not only a variegated group (or set of subgroups), but their makeup is changing rapidly. Meaningful roles need to be identified, programs developed, data obtained; and the right of access to resources of all kinds (including health and medical) means that those resources have to be available.

Major Concerns

When participants turned to the effort of identifying critical areas of concern which they felt to be central to the other problems discussed, three major areas emerged:

1. Methodologies of evaluating health, and concomitantly of evaluating health delivery systems and programs.

2. Bureaucratization; i.e., how does the current organization of services facilitate and/or impede the delivery of health services; what would make for a more optimal system?

71

3. Education, affecting responsibilities, behavior, attitudes, perceptions, and expectations of providers (including decision makers) and of patients alike.

Value Statements

Working with the foregoing, the group tried to formulate several statements of values which should underlie and provide the basis for a social health care delivery system:

1. *Total health care is a right.* This includes not only the traditional modes of privacy and speciality medical/clinical care when necessary and appropriate, but all those other components discussed or alluded to earlier, including physical and mental health, education, prevention, and health maintenance, preferably on an ambulatory basis, and aimed at keeping patients functioning and well in their own homes, families, communities, or environments. This must extend beyond the "medical model" to an overall "health model," and preferably to a "social health system" in which recognition is given to the needs of the patients, particularly the elderly, for related components such as adequate income, housing, nutrition, security, social activity, leisure, and recreation, to name but the most obvious ones.

2. *Access to what is already in existence is a right*, as a corollary to the previous statement.

3. *Quality of life* is to be striven for, as contrasted with an emphasis purely upon the prolongation of life.

4. *The concepts of caring and coping (Dana) need to be stressed more than continued investments in already sophisticated technologic systems.* This was emphasized in a number of ways: the proportion of the GNP spent on personal health versus education or prevention; our dismal record as measured by health indices and escalating costs despite the vast amounts being spent on clinical and technologic services; and the historical fact that most improvements in public and social health have tended to parallel social and economic changes in society, often predating the more exciting and romantic clinical/technical research discoveries.

5. *Any new system must not follow the disease-medical model, but must emphasize the positives of social health* (e.g., to use people's strengths, educate for health maintenance, and the prevention of illness).

72

Implementation

In examining how to ensure the translation of these values into programs meeting the social health needs of the aged, the participants enunciated several further concerns and possible approaches:

1. This system of values places primary emphasis upon the continuity of care in the community, working with people's coping abilities, examining the present acute care delivery system quite critically, recognizing the importance of research and ensuring the provision of basic research, and looking at health education on a continuum for all segments of our society. This value stance and its implementation would of necessity mean that financial priorities would also have to shift. What this implies is that our workshop would propose, on the basis of our own value judgments, the shifting of major funds to areas from which they are currently being withheld or even withdrawn. This was felt to be an awesome and intergenerational task.

2. The health system in general might well learn from the pediatricians who, in a sense, were the originators of community medicine and ambulatory care concepts in this country, and who have tended to factor out the sicknesses of children as a clinical speciality, while fostering a health system based on growth, development, prevention, nutrition, education, and long-term primary care.

3. Training for a specialized body of knowledge is essential. This can be approached in a variety of ways, and needs a great deal of study and work. Social work training has not yet developed a sufficient body of knowledge with respect to the aging. In this area, the schools of social work have produced "managing agents," running people's lives.

In the United States, medicine tends to view geriatric medicine not as a speciality, but as an offshoot of general clinical medicine, applied to a particular age group, whose problems, be they physiologic, clinical, or social, are not seen as being essentially different from anyone else's. There *is* a tendency for this to change, with the preliminary establishment recently of geriatric programs in three or four of the New York City medical schools. The comment was made here that other countries, such as Great Britain and the Scandinavian nations, tend to consider geriatrics more in terms of "clinical gerontology," and may be decades ahead of us in this area, as has too often been true in other social health areas as well.

While the medical model has not worked well for geriatric social health needs, it was noted that, from the pragmatic point of view, the specialized body of pathophysiologic and clinical knowledge which is needed will not be developed unless there is relative specialization plus funding for research, education, and training. It is essential to have interlocking systems, and there is a need for a much greater curriculum content regarding the social/medical/health problems of the aging at all levels of education.

4. Following a somewhat different trend of thought, accessibility was defined functionally as ensuring that the various social health services would be readily available to the aged. Thus, for example, Health Maintenance Organizations (HMOs) should be fostered and strategically located so that an individual in need can readily get to a hospital or health care source, or alternatively, have the health care source get to the individual as needed.

This led to a brief debate relative to the rather sophisticated concept of an HMO. It was concluded that if there was neither accessibility *nor* availability, then there is no functional HMO and, for that given individual patient, there is no health care delivery system at all. Perhaps we are saying that a flexible network is needed: in the United States, unlike other nations, we have chosen an opposite course; i.e., the expansion of medical schools and centralized regional, specialized, tertiary care; we have not trained the system's staff and personnel to go out to the peoples or the communities.

Conclusions

Having spent the entire day deliberating and debating these weighty matters, often in a manner and direction which initially had not even been conceived of, the members of the workshop felt stimulated and challenged, yet drained and frustrated by the time the afternoon session drew to a close. There was a general feeling that a great *beginning* had been made; that a number of key issues which had been nagging at each of the participants individually had at least been brought to the surface, grappled with, verbalized, perhaps even personified as one of our personal "devils"; that ideas, conflicts, and issues had been chewed on and partially digested or rejected in a unique opportunity for cross-cultural and interdisciplinary give-and-take; some major concerns had been expressed; and some value statements verbalized.

The workshop's general recommendations may be summarized as follows:

1. There must be emphasis upon the preventive aspects of social health care;

2. In dealing with the aging, we must deal with the entire spectrum of life;

3. There needs to be an interlocking of the various sytems in society affecting the aging;

4. Research must be contiguous with efforts to meet the current ongoing needs of the aging.

5. Training, education, and research toward building a body of knowledge is crucial; thus, education at all levels, with all systems, and with various professions, and including a broad spectrum of society, is essential.

Gideon Horowitz, PH.D.
Brookdale Social Health Center for the Aging
Professor, Adelphi University
Visiting Professor of Community Medicine
Mount Sinai School of Medicine
City University of New York

John P. Maher, M.D., M.P.H.
Director, Ambulatory Care
and Clinical Director
Brookdale Social Health Center for the Aging
The Mount Sinai Hospital
Assistant Professor of Clinical Medicine
Mount Sinai School of Medicine
City University of New York

Reference

[1] This workshop was under the joint sponsorship of the Brookdale Social Health Center for the Aging at The Mount Sinai Hospital and The Doris Siegel Memorial Fund.

Part 3
Conclusions

Some Suggested Remedies, Resolutions, and Further Deliberations

SAMUEL J. BOSCH

HELEN REHR

HAROLD LEWIS

Can one ever conclude the deliberations on "ethics and values" in any system of care? Or will every view of what the professional stance "ought to be" at a given point in time conflict with what "is"?

The Doris Siegel Memorial Fund Colloquium opened with Victor Fuchs' paper which challenged us to seek the social policy reflecting value and ethical choices in health care delivery—the "common good." Bess Dana's paper bridged the gap from policy to practice, highlighting the issues governing the professional on behalf of "individual good," in the delivery of quality care. Throughout the two-day colloquium, these themes predominated with repeated evidence of the difficulty that exists for all professions and disciplines in reconciling the "common good" with the "individual good."

The formal Fuchs and Dana presentations were followed by remarkably interesting and provocative workshop discussions. Workshop participants evidenced a pragmatic and realistic concern for the issues posed, relating their discussions to the settings and actions most meaningful to them. The decision to include multi-professional and multidiscipline competencies in the workshops provided a means of sensitizing participants to the different perspectives of participating disciplines and professions, and to their differences in approaches to issues of ethics. When these experts addressed health care needs, they stated them in general terms:

needs of consumers
needs of providers
needs of society.

The participants struggled with a very difficult topic and with diversity of perception and opinion to issues of ethics. They welcomed the interaction and found the diversity stimulating. It was interesting that the participants felt that the colloquium had liberated them from notions about their own and other professions, and from their local biases. Meeting with others opened the doorway to

79

fresh ideas and possibilities. They immediately recognized the difference in perceptions and began to struggle with the issues, agreeing to disagree. In the exchanges that occurred, participants enumerated and ordered priorities, and sought to achieve specificity and relevance for action rather than in-depth analysis of the issues. Obviously, participants felt they could not prescribe ethical imperatives without first venting their own perceptions of the most troublesome questions they faced in their own specialities. They acknowledged openly that many factors over a long period of time had worked to undermine values and ethical behavior in health matters. Nevertheless, all knew of evidence in the one-to-one relationship between patient and provider and felt comfortable in dealing with values and ethics as expressed in that dimension.

As one grappled with the expressed content of the groups, one became more and more aware that all were addressing traditional ethical behavior—the ethos of medicine in storied Hippocratic terms. Most of the participants believed that professional codes of ethics govern the usual and ordinary encounter between practitioner and patient, i.e., when an individual in distress reaches out for professional assistance with the expectation of finding prescribed knowledge and skills. What they described was the "breakdown" or the "archaic state" of codes of ethics. They noted that there is an erosion of ethical behavior throughout our society. In health care, it is evidenced by the lack of trust by patients of their practitioners and by people of the institutions which serve them. All agreed that serious reappraisal of "ethics" is needed. All of the professions and disciplines address different professional "codes of ethics" representing the obligations perceived by the professions themselves. Under the assumption of social contract, these guilds have ascribed to themselves selectness and elitism and have functioned in self-autonomy and self-regulation in return for a commitment to the common good.

However, the plurality of values, the differences among people, class, cultures in contemporary society makes the concept of "common good" very difficult to attain. Dicta found in the Hippocratic oath, such as the rejection of abortion, of euthanasia, or of safeguarding the secrets of the "art" are in conflict with today's social situation. Individuals in stress, seeking care, call for humanistic values and find marked gaps in the behaviors of practitioners. Can we have a "practice success" but an "ethical failure"? The impact of new technologies and new knowledge in medical science has led most people to expect cures for their illnesses and the health care practitioners have given silent acquiescence to this expectation. Frequently the professional, wishing to advance his professional status, is unmindful of the general public benefit. Is he acting on behalf of the "professional good" when he reaches for newer therapies such as behavioral modification or genetic manipulation, which may have individual benefit but which, when viewed on behalf of the "common good," may create major public concerns?

"Does the means justify the ends?" was the question before the participants. New social values and new social movements have added to the conflict so that among women the "rightness" to abortion is debated, among families the "rightness" to prolongation of life versus euthanasia for terminally ill members is a moral struggle. In all of these struggles, the participants noted, there are also the personal values of the professional as well.

What emerged among all the working parties was that there is no ready reconciliation of the values relevant to the "individual good" and those relevant to the "common good." There was agreement that a humanistic ethical relationship between practitioner and patient must be recovered in today's health care delivery. Recommendations were made by the participants that the individual patient-provider ethic should continue, that it should be held in the shared understanding of renewed concepts of social contract, and that professions should continue to socialize their newcomers to their values by teaching those elements on a case-by-case basis. But most of the participants were much less secure and comfortable in making recommendations regarding the way health resources (human and material) interact in relation to the population as a whole. When they attempted to identify values on behalf of the common good, there were more differences than similarities in their projections. It was in dealing with the population as against individuals that the participants of one group reacted with more concern and uneasiness over the "significant" finding that the varied representation did not allow them to reach mutual understandings. Whether this reflected a need to defend each one's professional values, or an inability as yet to define values that cut across professions was not uncovered during the workshops.

In tackling the individual and social dimensions of health care there was recognition that the "state of the art" of professional practice needs to be taken into account as one seeks resolution of value and ethical dilemmas. There was full recognition that it is unrealistic today to expect any one practitioner to encompass all available knowledge and skills. The existing states of overcommitment were highlighted. There was agreement that probably different types of interrelated practitioners, practices, and services, a sort of regional network of resources, should be required to assume responsibility for maintaining the health of defined population groups. There was no question that a great deal is needed in order to reconcile the differences among the health care providers alone; that the professions will need a clearer understanding of goals, values, and competencies of each other in order to secure quality collaboration.

When projections were made about what should be done to remedy the health care system of today, it was interesting that almost all supported the general benefit of pluralism. While there was recognition that the existing monolithic health systems in other countries were coming up with better health indicators, most participants wished to modify rather than to scrap the possibility of freedom of choice for both consumers and providers. There was agreement that we could develop a rational health care program under an authoritarian political system but the cost to us could be overwhelming. If we agree to settle for a democracy, then we may also need to settle for faltering, conflicting steps on a rocky road to planning and ultimate policy. Many seemed to agree that it is possible to negotiate social improvement in a capitalistic system both to provide an adequate care program and to enable professionals and health care workers to earn their livings in caring for people. They agreed that they were not addressing a profit motive but rather seeking a better distribution of power and a reorganization of incentives to assure both benefits to consumer and provider satisfaction; in short, they were urgently seeking effectiveness and effiiciency along with accountability of the provider to the consumer.

Numerous remedies and recommendations were made within the context of minimal expectations which are in themselves value-laden for a health care system. In-depth discussions of all such issues would have required much more time than was available. But at least all agreed that the future called for more than a "health care system" and guidelines for a broad social health system began to be prescribed. In essence, with good will and imagination, we have been able to draw from the discussions the following guidelines for social health care services, for education, and for research:

a. There should be universal access to health care based on basic population needs and on securing optimum social functioning.
b. There should be mutual participation of consumers and providers in policy making and in the operation of programs, with accountability of the provider to the consumer.
c. There should be an element of choice for consumers from among many options of care.
d. Availability and comprehensiveness of care should be guaranteed within reasonable distances, timely, and within community needs.
e. Human and material health resources should be reorganized in regionalized networks based on population needs.
f. There should be an element of predictability in program budgets.
g. Physicians should do doctoring at the primary, secondary, and tertiary levels, but in partnership with a broad range of manpower from other disciplines, and with differential manpower overseen by professionals.
h. Preventive actions and health education both for individuals and populations should be given high priority. Prevention incentives should be incorporated.
i. All health care professionals should be educated to function in a social health care system.
j. Educational goals should address a concept of bio-social psychological care, health maintenance, and prevention.
k. Education should be broadened to include the learning of interprofessional appreciation and collaboration.
l. Research cannot be limited to the basic sciences, but needs to include clinical and community health services as well.

But these are only the emerging guidelines that *we* have been able to detect from the content of the discussions. There were obviously many others, highly diverse in nature but directed toward innovative forms of service delivery, always in an open, freedom-of-choice system. Their diversity made it difficult to claim them as "group opinion." The interdependence of systems was constantly referred to, recognizing that caring and services could have their locus in any system, even outside that of the traditional medical establishment, and could be a method by which needs and resources could be meaningfully dealt with. Because the social health problem was identified as broader than medical, it was felt that the study of medicine does not prepare its practitioners for the broader responsibility. The money, the planning, and the policies need to be directed toward overall social health issues, rather than medical issues alone.

In addition, lessons derived from the colloquium were suggestive for future work on the theme of values and ethical dilemmas in relation to social health care:

a. It is apparent that the major product of the workshops, excluding the personal benefits the participants may have experienced, is the series of questions on values and ethics formulated by attendees. In all ways, their questions advanced from those they started with.

b. It seems that an effective way to identify value and ethical dilemmas in their most useful form is to provide the professionals who must live with them in practice an opportunity to express their concerns. The colloquium, in providing such an opportunity through its format—particularly in the inclusion of a number of professions and disciplines—achieved this unintended yet useful consequence.

c. The sequence was reiterated in all workshops, which apparently anticipates the learning pattern of participants and suggests an educational strategy for those interested in teaching ethics for practice.

Assuming that key concepts are sufficiently clear so all communicate with common meanings, learners must be informed initially about the form and content, structure and function, goals and methods, that constitute the practice under study. Then issues that arise in that practice involving choices in ambiguous situations should be identified, and their elements analyzed. Only when these two prerequisites have been mastered can a meaningful discussion of ethical issues inherent in such choices be undertaken, with the expectation that a deeper understanding of these ethical issues will result. It is also apparent that ignorance of the methodology that is employed in considering axiomatic questions hampers a full and productive analysis of these questions.

As professionals related to health we seem far more willing to discuss what *should* be our preferred behavior and that of the organizations with which we are associated, than we are willing to consider the collective welfare and our obligations for the common good. We appear to place individual need before collective need, and our focus on virtues and duties reflects this preference. Nevertheless, we seem to appreciate that many critical ethical concerns cannot be addressed in this order of preference; we seem to know

84

that many health service delivery ethical issues will not be resolved as long as this order of preference persists.

We are all agreed that ethical behavior is the foundation of professionalism. We are still limited, however, to the single case approach; our decisions are bioethical: e.g., prolongation of life or euthanasia for the *individual*. There is no doubt that humanistic commitments are the core minimum in professional-patient relationships in relation to the individual, but there needs to be preparation of tomorrow's health care professionals in social-professional ethics. They will need to be able to explore and to examine just and reasonable differences among issues and approaches so as to assure an improved equilibrium between the health care profession and society.

Samuel J. Bosch, M.D.
Associate Professor of Community Medicine
Mount Sinai School of Medicine
City University of New York

Helen Rehr, D.S.W.
Director, Department of Social Work Services
The Mount Sinai Hospital
Edith J. Baerwald Professor of Community Medicine (Social Work)
Mount Sinai School of Medicine
City University of New York

Harold Lewis, D.S.W.
Dean, Hunter College School of Social Work
City University of New York

Appendices

Doris Siegel Memorial Fund Committee

Honorary Chairmen

Thomas C. Chalmers, M.D.
   President, The Mount Sinai Medical Center
   Dean, Mount Sinai School of Medicine
   City University of New York

Kurt W. Deuschle, M.D.
   Ethel H. Wise Professor and Chairman
   Department of Community Medicine
   Mount Sinai School of Medicine
   City University of New York

S. David Pomrinse, M.D.
   Executive Vice President
   The Mount Sinai Medical Center
   Edmond A. Guggenheim Professor of Administrative Medicine
   Mount Sinai School of Medicine
   City University of New York

Hans Popper, M.D., PH.D.
   President Emeritus
   The Mount Sinai Medical Center
   Dean Emeritus and Gustave L. Levy Distinguished Service Professor
   Mount Sinai School of Medicine
   City University of New York

Committee

Mrs. Jack R. Aron
   Vice Chairman of the Board
   The Mount Sinai Medical Center

Arthur H. Aufses, Jr., M.D.
   Director of Surgery
   The Mount Sinai Hospital
   Chairman and Franz W. Sichel Professor
   Department of Surgery
   Mount Sinai School of Medicine
   City University of New York

Henry David Banta, M.D.
Research Director, Health Program
Office of Technology Assessment
Congress of the United States

Mrs. Robert M. Benjamin
Member of the Board
The Mount Sinai Medical Center

Philip Bernstein, M.S.S.A.
Executive Vice President
Council of Jewish Federations and Welfare Funds, Inc.

Samuel J. Bosch, M.D.
Associate Professor of Community Medicine
Mount Sinai School of Medicine
City University of New York

Bess Dana, M.S.S.A.
Associate Professor
Director, Education Unit
Department of Community Medicine
Mount Sinai School of Medicine
City University of New York

Richard Gorlin, M.D.
Chairman, Department of Medicine
The Mount Sinai Hospital
Murray M. Rosenberg Professor of Medicine
Mount Sinai School of Medicine
City University of New York

Gail Green Grob, M.S.W.
Preceptor, Department of Social Work Services
The Mount Sinai Hospital

Celia Moss Hailperin, M.S.W.

Jack Herman
Vice President for Development
The Mount Sinai Medical Center

Mrs. Walter A. Hirsch
Member of the Board
The Mount Sinai Medical Center

Kurt Hirschhorn, M.D.
Professor and Chairman
Department of Pediatrics
The Mount Sinai Hospital
Herbert H. Lehman Professor of Pediatrics
Mount Sinai School of Medicine
City University of New York

M. Ralph Kaufman, M.D.*
Esther and Joseph Klingenstein Professor of Psychiatry Emeritus
Dean Emeritus and Consultant to the Page & William Black Post-Graduate
    School of Medicine
Mount Sinai School of Medicine
City University of New York

Mrs. Seymour M. Klein
Member of the Board
The Mount Sinai Medical Center

Harold Lewis, D.S.W.
Dean, Hunter College School of Social Work
City University of New York

Robert D. London, M.D.*
Director of Ambulatory Care
The Mount Sinai Hospital
Professor of Clinical Pediatrics
Associate Professor of Community Medicine
Mount Sinai School of Medicine
City University of New York

Janice Paneth, M.S.
Associate Director, Department of Social Work Services
The Mount Sinai Hospital
Assistant Professor of Community Medicine
Mount Sinai School of Medicine
City University of New York

Beatrice Phillips, M.S.W.
Editor-in-Chief
Health and Social Work

Maurice V. Russell, ED.D.
Professor of Clinical Social Work and
Director of Social Service Department
New York University Medical Center

* Deceased

Marvin Stein, M.D.
  Director of Psychiatry
  The Mount Sinai Hospital
  Chairman and Esther and Joseph
    Klingenstein Professor
  Department of Psychiatry
  Mount Sinai School of Medicine
  City University of New York

Elinor Stevens, M.A.
  Senior Program Specialist
  Department of Standards and Accreditation
  Council on Social Work Education

Mrs. Frank L. Weil
  Member of the Board
  The Mount Sinai Medical Center

Executive Secretary

Helen Rehr, D.S.W.
  Director, Department of Social Work Services
  The Mount Sinai Hospital
  Edith J. Baerwald Professor of Community Medicine (Social Work)
  Mount Sinai School of Medicine
  City University of New York

Doris Siegel Memorial Colloquium Subcommittee on Planning

Mrs. Jack R. Aron

Mrs. Robert M. Benjamin

Samuel J. Bosch, M.D.*

Bess Dana, M.S.S.A.*

Mr. Jack Herman

Mrs. Seymour M. Klein

Harold Lewis, D.S.W.*

Beatrice Phillips, M.S.W.*

Helen Rehr, D.S.W.*

Maurice Russell, ED.D.*

Mrs. Elinor Stevens, M.A.*

Mrs. Frank L. Weil

Staff to the Committee

Mrs. Marjorie Pleshette, B.A.

*Subcommittee on program planning

APPENDIX C

Participants

Henry David Banta, M.D.
   Research Director, Health Program
   Office of Technology Assessment
   Congress of the United States

Patricia Bauman, M.S.
   Professional Staff Member
   Senate Committee on Human Resources

Barbara Berkman, D.S.W.
   Adjunct Assistant Professor of Community Medicine
   Mount Sinai School of Medicine
   City University of New York

L. Diane Bernard, PH.D.
   Dean, School of Social Work
   Florida State University

Richard H. Bernstein, M.D.
   Medical Director
   Group Health Plan of New Jersey

Samuel W. Bloom, PH.D.
   Professor of Sociology and Community Medicine
   Mount Sinai School of Medicine
   City University of New York

Werner W. Boehm, PH.D.
   Professor of Social Work
   Director, Center for International Comparative Social Welfare
   Rutgers University

Barbara Borden, M.S.
   Social Work Coordinator
   Visiting Nurse Service of New York

Abba E. Borowich, M.D.
   Senior Clinical Instructor of Psychiatry
   Mount Sinai School of Medicine
   City University of New York

Samuel J. Bosch, M.D.
: Associate Professor of Community Medicine
  Mount Sinai School of Medicine
  City University of New York

Ann Brancato, M.A.
: Director, Center for Aging
  Bronx Community College
  City University of New York

Minerva Brown, M.S.S.W.
: Director, The Page & William Black Post-Graduate School of Medicine
  Mount Sinai School of Medicine
  City University of New York

Catherine Caicedo, M.S.
: Assistant Professor
  New York University School of Social Work

Marjorie Cantor, M.S.
: Director, Research, Planning and Evaluation
  Office of the Mayor of New York City
  Department for the Aging

Phyllis Caroff, D.S.W.
: Professor
  Hunter College School of Social Work
  City University of New York

Thomas C. Chalmers, M.D.
: President, The Mount Sinai Medical Center
  Dean, Mount Sinai School of Medicine
  City University of New York

Beatrice Chase, ED.D.
: Consultant in Nursing
  New York

Roslyn Chernesky, D.S.W.
: Assistant Professor
  School of Social Work
  Columbia University

Sylvia S. Clarke, M.S.
: Director, Social Work Department
  The Roosevelt Hospital

Joan Bonner Conway, D.S.W.
Director, Department of Social Work
Hospital of The University of Pennsylvania

Raymond Cornbill, M.B.A.
Vice President, Planning and Management Information Systems
The Mount Sinai Medical Center

Bess Dana, M.S.S.A.
Associate Professor
Director, Education Unit
Department of Community Medicine
Mount Sinai School of Medicine
City University of New York

Marionette S. Daniels, M.S.W., A.C.S.W.
Instructor and Coordinator for Community Program Planning and
   Development of Community Medicine
Mount Sinai School of Medicine
City University of New York

Margaret A. Dennis, M.S.
Visiting Associate Professor
School of Social Welfare
State University of New York, Albany

Kurt W. Deuschle, M.D.
Ethel H. Wise Professor and Chairman
Department of Community Medicine
Mount Sinai School of Medicine
City University of New York

Rose Dobrof, D.S.W.
Associate Professor
Hunter College School of Social Work
City University of New York

Golda M. Edinburg, A.C.S.W.
Director, Social Work Department
McLean Hospital

Samuel K. Elster, M.D.
Clinical Professor of Medicine
Dean, The Page & William Black Post-Graduate School of Medicine
Associate Dean for Continuous Education
Mount Sinai School of Medicine
City University of New York

David E. Epperson, PH.D.
  Dean, Graduate School of Social Work
  University of Pittsburgh

Hans S. Falck, PH.D.
  Regenstein Professor of Social Services
  The Menninger Foundation

Ruth Fizdale, M.S.W.
  Executive Director
  Arthur Lehman Counseling Service

Irvin L. Foutz, M.S.W.
  Adjunct Associate Professor
  Graduate School of Social Work
  University of Pittsburgh

Harry Frankfurt, PH.D.
  Professor, Department of Philosophy
  Yale University

Phyllis B. Freeman, D.S.W.
  Assistant Professor
  Director of Doctoral Admissions
  Graduate School of Social Work
  University of Pennsylvania

Victor R. Fuchs, PH.D.
  Director
  Center for Economic Analysis of Human Behavior and Social Institutions
  Stanford, California

Harold Hepworth Gardner, M.D.
  Executive Director, Health Care Institute
  Wayne State University

Pearl S. German, SC.D.
  Director of Community Studies
  Johns Hopkins University

Donald B. Giddon, D.M.D., PH.D.
  Dean, College of Dentistry
  New York University

Mitchell I. Ginsberg, M.S.
  Dean, School of Social Work
  Columbia University

Stanley J. Goldsmith, M.D.
Assistant Professor of Physics/Nuclear Medicine
and Chairman of the Department
Mount Sinai School of Medicine
City University of New York

Harry M. Gordon, M.D.
Professor of Pediatrics
Albert Einstein College of Medicine

Gail Green Grob, M.S.W.
Preceptor, Department of Social Work Services
The Mount Sinai Hospital

Betty Gumpertz, M.S.W., A.C.S.W.
Director of Social Service
Beth Israel Hospital, Boston

Celia Moss Hailperin, M.S.W.
Member, Doris Siegel Memorial Committee

Emanuel Hallowitz, M.S.W.
Director of Social Service
Professor, Division of Biological Sciences and School of Social Services
Administration
University of Chicago

David Harris, M.D., M.P.H.
Commissioner
Suffolk County Department of Health Services

Rose Muscatine Hauer, R.N.
Director, Nursing Service & School of Nursing
Beth Israel Medical Center, New York

Jack Hirsch, D.D.S.
Assistant Clinical Professor of Dentistry
Mount Sinai School of Medicine
City University of New York

Gideon Horowitz, PH.D.
Brookdale Social Health Center for the Aging
Professor, Adelphi University
Visiting Professor of Community Medicine
Mount Sinai School of Medicine
City University of New York

Abraham Horwitz, M.D.
   Scholar in Residence
   Fogarty International Center
   National Institutes of Health

Marian H. Hosford, PH.D.
   Dean, School of Nursing
   The City College
   City University of New York

Linbania Jacobson, ED.D.
   Chief, Division of Health Behavior
   American Health Foundation

Barbara J. Johnson, M.S.
   Social Work Consultant
   Arthur C. Logan Hospital
   Deputy Chairperson, Africana Studies
   Brooklyn College

Mo Katz
   Deputy Director, Policy and Program Development
   Montefiore Hospital and Medical Center

Toba Schwaber Kerson, D.S.W.
   Assistant Professor
   The Graduate School of Social Work and Social Research
   Bryn Mawr College

Irving Ladimer, S.J.D.
   Adjunct Associate Professor of Community Medicine
   Mount Sinai School of Medicine
   City University of New York

Sybil H. Landau, LL.D.
   Associate Professor and Assistant Dean
   Benjamin N. Cardozo School of Law

Aaron Levenstein, J.D.
   Professor, Department of Management
   Baruch College
   City University of New York

Isaac Levi, PH.D.
   Professor, Department of Philosophy
   Columbia University

100

Harold Lewis, D.S.W.
    Dean, Hunter College School of Social Work
    City University of New York

Hannah Lipsky, M.S.
    Assistant Director
    Department of Social Work Services
    The Mount Sinai Hospital
    Instructor in Community Medicine
    Mount Sinai School of Medicine
    City University of New York

Harold Lipton, M.S., A.C.S.W.
    Director, Social Service
    Children's Hospital Medical Center
    Akron, Ohio

Helen Lokshin, M.S.
    Director, Social Service
    Elmhurst Hospital
    Assistant Professor of Community Medicine
    Mount Sinai School of Medicine
    City University of New York

Abraham Lurie, PH.D.
    Director, Social Work Services
    Long Island Jewish-Hillside Medical Center

Albert Lyons, M.D.
    Archivist
    The Mount Sinai Medical Center
    Clinical Professor of Surgery
    Mount Sinai School of Medicine
    City University of New York

Michael G. Macdonald, LL.D.
    Vice President and General Counsel
    The Mount Sinai Medical Center

John P. Maher, M.D., M.P.H.
    Director, Ambulatory Care
    and Clinical Director
    Brookdale Social Health Center for the Aging
    The Mount Sinai Hospital
    Assistant Professor of Clinical Medicine
    Mount Sinai School of Medicine
    City University of New York

Mildred D. Mailick, M.S.
Assistant Professor
Hunter College School of Social Work
City University of New York

Mannuccio Mannucci, M.D.
Associate Professor of Psychiatry
Mount Sinai School of Medicine
City University of New York

Neil McCluskey, PH.D.
Director, Office of Gerontological Studies
City University of New York Graduate School

Helen Cassidy McGrail, M.S.W.
Professor and Coordinator of Field Instruction
School of Social Work
Tulane University

Laura R. Merker, R.N., M.P.H.
Associate Director of Nursing
The Mount Sinai Hospital
Instructor in Community Medicine
Mount Sinai School of Medicine
City University of New York

Rosalind S. Miller, M.S.W.
Associate Professor
School of Social Work
Columbia University

Harry R. Moody, PH.D.
Executive Secretary
Brookdale Center on Aging of Hunter College
City University of New York

Joan E. Morgenthau, M.D.
Director of Adolescent Health Center
The Mount Sinai Hospital
Assistant Dean of Student Affairs for Clinical Years
and Associate Professor of Clinical Community Medicine
Mount Sinai School of Medicine
City University of New York

Elizabeth Murphy, R.N.
Assistant Director of Nursing
The Mount Sinai Hospital

Grace Neill, M.S.W.
  Preceptor, Department of Social Work Services
  The Mount Sinai Hospital

Janice Paneth, M.S.
  Associate Director, Department of Social Work Services
  The Mount Sinai Hospital
  Assistant Professor of Community Medicine
  Mount Sinai School of Medicine
  City University of New York

Beatrice Phillips, M.S.W.
  Editor-in-Chief
  Health and Social Work

S. David Pomrinse, M.D.
  Executive Vice President
  The Mount Sinai Medical Center
  Edmond A. Guggenheim Professor of Administrative Medicine
  Mount Sinai School of Medicine
  City University of New York

Ruth Ravich
  Coordinator, Patient Service Representative Program
  The Mount Sinai Hospital

Jeanette Regensburg, PH.D.
  Lecturer in Community Medicine
  Mount Sinai School of Medicine
  City University of New York

Helen Rehr, D.S.W.
  Director, Department of Social Work Services
  The Mount Sinai Hospital
  Edith J. Baerwald Professor of Community Medicine (Social Work)
  Mount Sinai School of Medicine
  City University of New York

Stanley Reichman, M.D.
  Director, Department of Community Medicine
  Hospital for Joint Diseases and Medical Center
  Assistant Professor of Community Medicine
  Mount Sinai School of Medicine
  City University of New York

Gary Rosenberg, PH.D.
Associate Director, Department of Social Work Services
The Mount Sinai Hospital
Assistant Professor of Community Medicine
Mount Sinai School of Medicine
City University of New York

Sidney D. Rosoff, J.D.
President, Society for the Right to Die

Maurice V. Russell, ED.D.
Professor of Clinical Social Work and
Director of Social Service Department
New York University Medical Center

James Satterwhite, M.S.
Director, Office of Staff Development and Training
Human Resources Administration
New York, New York

David Schonholz, M.D.
Associate Clinical Professor of Obstetrics/Gynecology
Mount Sinai School of Medicine
City University of New York

Gary B. Seltzer, M.S.S.W.
Behavioral Education Projects
Harvard University

Ruth K. Seltzer, M.S.W.
Director, Department of Social Work
Beth Israel Hospital, New York
Assistant Professor of Community Medicine
Mount Sinai School of Medicine
City University of New York

Lois Shein, M.S.W.
Preceptor, Department of Social Work Services
The Mount Sinai Hospital

Robert S. Siffert, M.D.
Professor of Orthopaedics and Chairman of the Department
Mount Sinai School of Medicine
City University of New York

Barbara Silverstone, D.S.W.
Chief of Social Services
Jewish Home and Hospital for Aged

104

Edward J. Speedling, M.A.
Research Associate
Quality Assurance—Nursing
The Mount Sinai Hospital

Roberta R. Spohn
Deputy Commissioner
New York City Department for the Aging

Carole J. Stapleton, M.S.
Senior Planning Analyst
The Mount Sinai Medical Center

Elinor Stevens, M.A.
Council on Social Work Education

Joseph A. Stewart, M.A.
Director, Cooperative Care Center
New York University Medical Center

Elaine T. Vayda, M.S.W.
Assistant Professor
McMaster University School of Social Work

Ramon Velez, M.D.
Assistant Professor of Medicine and Community Health Services
Duke University Medical Center

Patricia Volland, M.S.
Director, Department of Social Work
Johns Hopkins Hospital

Hyman J. Weiner, D.S.W.
Dean, Graduate School of Social Work
New York University

Gail Kuhn Weissman, R.N.
Associate Director, Inpatient Services
Director of Nursing
The Mount Sinai Hospital
Assistant Professor of Administrative Medicine
Mount Sinai School of Medicine
City University of New York

Moshe Yehuda, M.P.A.
Director for Organization and Administration
Kupat Holim
Histadrut, Tel Aviv

Alma T. Young, M.S.W.
  Assistant Director, Department of Social Work Services
  The Mount Sinai Hospital
  Instructor in Community Medicine
  Mount Sinai School of Medicine
  City University of New York

Ruth E. Zambrana, M.A.
  Senior Associate Sociologist
  Mount Sinai School of Medicine
  City University of New York

Ann Zimmer, M.S.
  Chairman, Task Force on Aging
  American Public Health Association

Gary Zucker, M.D.
  Chief, Division of Internal Medicine
  Beth Israel Medical Center, New York
  Clinical Professor of Medicine
  Mount Sinai School of Medicine
  City University of New York

Workshop Leaders

Phyllis Caroff, D.S.W.

Ruth Fizdale, M.S.W.

Gideon Horowitz, PH.D.

Abraham Lurie, PH.D.

Mildred D. Mailick, M.S.

Rosalind S. Miller, M.S.W.

Gary Rosenberg, PH.D.

APPENDIX E

Recorders

Catherine Caicedo, M.S.

Roslyn Chernesky, D.S.W.

Grace Neill, M.S.W.

Ruth K. Seltzer, M.S.W.

Edward J. Speedling, M.A.

Alma T. Young, M.S.W.

Ruth E. Zambrana, M.A.